Expecting Jewish!

A Millenial Mom's Practical Guide to
How Judaism Can be a Blessing
to new Moms and Moms-to-be

Marion Haberman

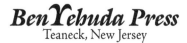
Teaneck, New Jersey

Published by Ben Yehuda Press
122 Ayers Court #1B
Teaneck, NJ 07666

http://www.BenYehudaPress.com

To subscribe to our monthly book club and support independent Jewish publishing, visit https://www.patreon.com/BenYehudaPress

Ben Yehuda Press books may be purchased at a discount by synagogues, book clubs, and other institutions buying in bulk. For information, please email markets@BenYehudaPress.com

Cover illustration by Laura Bradford (www.lcbradfordart.com)

Permissions and Acknowledgements:

ISBN13 978-1-934730-84-3

21 22 23 / 10 9 8 7 6 5 4 3 2 1   20210205

Dedication

To my baby boys, who inspired me to write this book. I think about each of you each day, whether I get to hold you in my arms or just in my heart. You will always be the best part of me.

To my husband, Andrew. You supported me unconditionally through every part of this process. Your encouragement was unwavering and your enthusiasm lifted me up when I felt defeated. You are my sunshine in the rain.

To my family, thank you for being some of my first interviewees and social media followers. When I told you about my ideas I shared them with a hint of a question mark, but you answered with an exclamation point and made me believe I could do it.

And to all the moms in my life who have shown me the way: Patsy, Lesley, Vickey, Hannah, Maude, Susie, Donna and Gloria. Thank you.

Contents

Introduction

There are two words that come to mind when I think about bringing a child into this world: wonder and miracle. Giving birth, or witnessing one, is the single closest experience a person can have to the very act of creation. I remember the first few moments right after my first son was born. I held him on my chest and thought how strange this all was. Just a few moments beforehand, he had been just as he was then, but within me; and then he was a living breathing person all on his own. The wonder in all of this is overpowering; no matter how much science we learn about the process, the miracle of it will never cease to amaze. But if you're reading this you're probably more concerned about when to send out a bris invite and you don't have time to ruminate on wonders and miracles! So let's jump in.

This book is a practical guide to pregnancy, through a Jewish lens. When you're expecting a baby and you're Jewish there are all sorts of ways in which Jewish tradition, faith and culture can be a blessing to you. This book is broken down into trimesters and provides a guide for how to both incorporate and benefit from including Judaism in your pregnancy journey. I wrote this book to answer the questions I received about what to do during all the stages of pregnancy from women whose upbringing, rabbis or communities weren't giving them an easy answer. My hope is that this book will be a helpful one-stop shop for relatable, practical and spiritual advice.

When I got pregnant I found myself consumed by the minutiae of preparing for a baby: What was the best car seat to buy? Should I register for onesies with buttons or zippers (zippers, always go for zippers!)? These things literally kept me up at night. I also found myself daydreaming about the first Jewish aspects of my son's life, like his bris.

I imagined it would be this dreamlike calm and happy celebration where the closest people in my life would come to welcome my baby into this world. As my due date got closer I realized I actually had never planned anything like a bris and had no idea where to start. How and when was I supposed to invite people? Did people send out invitation emails from the delivery room? I went on YouTube (my trusted source for peer-to-peer information) hoping to see tons of videos on the topic, just like the millions there are about *What to Pack in your Hospital Delivery Bag* (search *that* on YouTube if you'd like spend the next 10 hours of your day watching people unpack and repack their hospital bags while describing in detail why they chose each item).

I was disappointed to see my search box come up blank. There were some videos explaining a bris from religious organizations like Chabad, and other factual content from BimBam; but there were no *real* moms giving personal "I just lived through it so let me tell you how it is" advice.

Six months later I gave birth to my baby boy, and semi-successfully planned a crazy, emotional, overwhelming, beautiful 80-person bris and I thought, I'm going to share my experience online. And that's how my YouTube Channel, *MyJewishMommyLife* was born.

When I began to share my journey to motherhood online, I was surprised to learn how many other Jewish moms had experiences similar to my own. There's this myth that Judaism doesn't play a role in preparing for a baby until the baby is actually born, because there are limited Jewish rituals and obligations for women during this time in their lives. Sandy Falk and Rabbi Daniel Judson explain in their book, *The Jewish Pregnancy Book*: "(the) Talmudic Rabbis, who formulated the basis of traditional Jewish prayer, ritual and law, were men, so they never experienced pregnancy. As a result, there are a dearth of prayers, rituals and blessings that Judaism has for pregnancy and delivery."

Creating a family is one of the most significant aspects of Judaism; yet, most Jewish life cycle books only begin with the very first Jewish ceremony—the *brit milah*, or baby naming. This is a little strange; even if you believe life begins at birth, how can it be that a religion that celebrates every moment of life has nothing to say about becoming pregnant?

And what is a nice Jewish girl to do when she gets pregnant? Rabbi Shira Stutman of 6th and I Synagogue in Washington, D.C. explained to me that some Jewish people are so superstitious; it often happens that the experience of being pregnant and Jewish is more about what you *don't* do. In addition, Jewish law does not consider a baby to have a life of its own until it's born. Before that, it is just part of the gestational carrier's body, which results in ritual around Jewish pregnancy being "complicated." In the seventeenth and eighteenth centuries, a collection of prayers called *tkhines* (Yiddish for *supplications*) introduced a codified text of prayers and private poems intended for women and home life. So while there's a historic precedence for including a spiritual component to the physical experience of pregnancy and childbirth, today these ancient *tkhines* prayers are not widely known outside of ultra-Orthodox circles.

Today there is a movement within the Jewish community to honor the mother's role in conception and giving birth and to celebrate the spiritual component of pregnancy. Even with 4,000 years of ritual behind us, there's still some catching up to do! Women are writing their own prayers for those most difficult and painful moments that occur in childbirth and pregnancy. Today there are web sites like RitualWell.org, where Jewish women contribute new thoughts, prayers and poems to a growing collection. Jewish birth workers and doulas are also sharing their techniques and practices for incorporating Jewish spirituality into childbirth, and female communities like those that gather in Well Circles organized by At The Well are talking more and more about how important this is for the mental health of new moms.

This movement is seizing the opportunity for women to create their own rituals to make up for the lack of traditional Jewish customs and experiences around pregnancy. Women are taking agency and creating and adapting tradition to their needs. In this book I expand on the traditional offerings of halachic Judaism and include old and new ways in which Jewish women are incorporating their Judaism into their pregnancies.

Generally though, even a woman who is fairly religious and participates in Jewish life and the Jewish community will not experience a formal connection between Judaism and pregnancy until she gives birth. I began researching this because it just didn't make sense to me that such a crucial and fruitful nine months of a woman's life could be so barren of spiritual connection. I always thought that Judaism would have a ton to say about pregnancy, as it generally does about almost everything else. And just as there are hundreds of different strollers I didn't yet know about, I assumed I would learn about the hundreds of things I needed to know about Judaism and pregnancy in the same way. I was confused and frustrated to learn that there wasn't a wealth of information easily available. That's why I wrote *Expecting Jewish*—to highlight how rich this tradition can be when it comes to pregnancy.

I started collecting stories from friends and relatives on their experiences with childbirth as a Jewish person and set out to create a handbook of Jewish pregnancy. While every pregnant woman seems to own another pregnancy handbook—*What to Expect when You're Expecting*—no one seemed to have a Jewish pregnancy handbook close at hand. My goal is to change that.

From conception to birth, this book is a how-to guide that focuses on preparing for motherhood from a Jewish perspective. It covers everything from the practicalities of planning a *bris* to the mysticism of the *mikvah*. This book shares an unfiltered perspective on what to really expect during this stage of life, with advice from real moms who have lived through it. Interviews with rabbis and social media game-changers in the Jewish community also offer insight on what's trending and what's changing for Jewish women today when it comes to forsaking superstitions and embracing a powerful feminine role in motherhood.

This book also includes interviews with rabbis and Jewish community leaders who are, in very personal ways, leading the charge and offering a new perspective on how synagogues and Jewish communities can be more welcoming and helpful to pregnant women.

Oh, and before we dive in, let's start with the #1 question (according to many rabbis!) that Jewish pregnant women have: Do you need to fast on Yom Kippur? Short answer: *NO!* Jewish laws always prioritize life, called *pikuach nefesh*; and because it would be dangerous for the baby and mom to fast (while pregnant and breastfeeding), a woman is not obligated to do so.

The Jewish Pregnancy Checklist

Here is a short checklist to keep on hand throughout your pregnancy. Use it when you feel lost in this long nine-month journey as a means to center yourself once again and find comfort and inspiration from your Jewish tradition. You will find an expanded explanation of everything in this list throughout the book.

1st Trimester Checklist
- ❑ Decide when you want to share the news that you're expecting, who you'd like to tell and how you'd like to tell them.
- ❑ Research, discuss and decide on what genetic testing you want to have done.
- ❑ Reserve your internal resources and reflections for self-care; consider immersing in the mikvah.
- ❑ Start enjoying Couples' Shabbat.

2nd Trimester Checklist
- ❑ Think about how to you'd like to make your birth experience positive and your own.
- ❑ Write down what being a good Jewish parent means to you and what's a priority for your growing family.
- ❑ Research options for new mom groups, Jewish baby classes, synagogue community, etc.
- ❑ Try Jewish meditation as a way to calm and soothe yourself and prepare for labor and delivery.

3rd Trimester Checklist
- ❑ Start to narrow down an English and Hebrew baby name.
- ❑ Think about how you'd like to nourish your baby (both physically and spiritually).
- ❑ If you're having a boy, figure out who you would like to attend the bris and where you will hold it. Find and reach out to a

mohel and let them know when you are due.

- ❏ Immerse in the mikvah.
- ❏ Give tzedakah either through financial donation or time.
- ❏ Create a spiritual birth plan.
- ❏ Find out if your synagogue organizes a meal train or other support services for new parents. If they don't, talk to your friends and family about how you'd like them to support you when the baby arrives.

4th Trimester
- ❏ Rest.
- ❏ First Shabbat as a new family.
- ❏ Have a bris for your son or baby naming for your daughter.
- ❏ Put up a mezuzah in your baby's nursery.
- ❏ Download Jewish children's music.

Expecting Jewish!

Before Everything Begins

I.

Sacred Kosher Sex and Finding Out You're Pregnant

I've often been curious about this idea: if you knew you were going to conceive on a certain attempt, would you have sex a different way? I'm not talking about positions per se, but would you try to be more sensual, more giving, more loving? There's an ancient Jewish legend that for a woman to conceive a son (males were preferred in those times) she needs to orgasm before her partner. That's a nice thought. Judaism has a lot to say about kosher sex because, after all, it's a mitzvah! So let's start with the art of sacred sex; because after all, this *is* how babies are made.

Have you ever felt that instant connection to someone you've only just met? In Judaism, that's not rare. In Jewish mysticism there's a story that when a person is born they are assigned a letter in the Torah. It might just be the letter Bet that begins the whole Bible with the word '*bereysheet*' (in the Beginning); or maybe it's just in the middle part of a word in some lesser-known chapter. The legend goes something like this: Two people who feel that immediate affection toward one another likely have letters on the same page or in the same section of the Torah as their own. And, if you're really lucky, and find someone whose letter is in the same sentence or even word as yours, then you've just met your soulmate. Mazal tov! In Judaism, the journey from love to conception is not just a physical act. There's a role for God and fate here, too.

In Judaism women are often regarded as being more spiritual than men. Men are required to observe additional mitzvot: They wrap tefillin and wear tzitzit to raise themselves up to the spiritual plane that women already inhabit. In the same way, women are also considered more sexual than men. In her book, *The Voice of Sarah*, Tamar Frankel suggests that these two conceptions of a woman's identity are inherently paradoxical but also complementary—that there is some connection between sensuality and spirituality. The Torah is full of stories of women using their divinely ordained sensual power to seduce men (beginning with Eve and her tempting apple!), and continuing on with other writings like the story of Queen Esther, the heroine of Purim who seduced a king and used her influence over him to save the Jewish people. So...what have you used your sensual powers for lately?

However you want to interpret these core components of our folklore, for me the key takeaway is that Judaism has always understood that sexuality—especially the female side of it—has great power. This innate component of our identity is the foundation of conception and is something to celebrate.

What's love (and God) got to do with it?

Judaism recognizes the concept of a soulmate—*beshert* in Yiddish. The word *beshert* means fate, destiny, or the idea that something or someone is destined and "meant to be." The idea of finding your *beshert* holds a lot of meaning in the Jewish community. It's used as a kind phrase when things don't work out—"it wasn't *beshert*"—and reminds us that as humans we sometimes need to surrender to elements of life that are beyond our control. The word *beshert* also connotes "God's will" or "from God." The term *beshert* is also used as a form of shorthand for the person you're going to marry. You may have been asked if you've met your *beshert* yet.

Judaism also has a love of matchmaking. The role of a *shadkhan*, or professional matchmaker, is still a revered and respected part of Jewish society, especially in modern religious communities. Even the ancient rabbis were concerned with who married whom. The Torah begins with a long lineage list of generations (was this perhaps the first gossip column or *NYTimes* Wedding section?). Aside from Eve, who was created for Adam, the stories in the Torah go into great detail about how each matriarch and patriarch found one another.

Abraham sought a wife for his son Isaac by sending out a servant to find her. Jacob worked for Leah and Rachel's father for many years in order to be worthy of them. Many times these biblical journeys for love are filled with trials and trepidations along the way. Woven throughout these epic tales are instances both of God's intervention as well as individual assertion. Our tradition is built on these examples of finding companionship and love.

One interesting thought on the concept of a soulmate in Judaism is that although it is ordained in heaven and perhaps beyond our free will, there is no guarantee of a good marriage just because the union is with your soulmate. That's where it's up to each of us to put forth the effort and commitment to create a happy union.

Jewish tradition, aside from the notions of *beshert*, are very clear on the commitment and approach required to keeping couples together. In the first book of the Torah, Beresheet, it is written, "Then the Lord God said, 'it is not good for man to be alone'" (Genesis 2:18). Many of the Jewish laws and requirements about family life are designed to keep families together and to give children a solid foundation and home environment. Today there are many Jewish writings that reimagine the idea of *beshert* as something you and your partner continue to create as you reinvest in your relationship and build it together.

So, is love created by God or by man? The religious scholar Simon Jacobson answers: Both! In his article 'Marriage: Destiny or Chance?' he writes, "Like everything in life, we are partners with God in creation. The Divine sends each soul off on its unique journey through life, and designates which soul belong with another. But we humans, through our choices and actions, can change the course for the better (and also, sadly, for the worse)."

Time to be fruitful

So you've found your *beshert* and you've decided to be fruitful and multiply. What's the first Jewish step to take?

Many doctors today will recommend a pre-pregnancy checkup to see if your body is ready and healthy enough to have a baby. They may recommend gaining or losing weight, adjusting your diet and exercise—and they'll almost definitely recommend the woman to start taking a prenatal vitamin every day. I would suggest that it's not a bad idea for a couple to do a relationship pre-pregnancy checkup as well. Is everything healthy with the relationship? Do both partners feel equally supported? Are you both on the same page about having children and what the future of caring for that child will look like? Beyond the physical and relationship assessment for the couple, it's also important to do an 'emotional' check up on yourself. Have you taken care of yourself in a way that has made you strong enough to now care for someone else?

I asked Rabbi Sara Brandes, Executive Director at Or HaLev: Center for Jewish Spirituality and Meditation, about the spiritual connection between God and women. She shared with me that Judaism has a complicated relationship with the fact that women bring children into the world through their bodies. In one capacity, there is tremendous respect for the feminine ability to create life, but there can also be secrecy and shame when a woman experiences infertility. The primary way this plays out, ritually speaking, is through the mikvah, the ritual bath—which is outside of regular synagogue life.

Although there is no obligation to immerse in the mikvah once you are pregnant, there is a Jewish law that women should visit the mikvah after giving birth. Rabbi Sara told me that unlike the pregnancy app on your phone, Judaism isn't really there for the weekly play by play; there aren't rituals or prayers to say when your baby goes from the size of an avocado to a pineapple. But, there is a tremendous spiritual connection that women can have to God and to Judaism during this time, and a mikvah immersion can be part of that.

In terms of self-care, you may want to visit the mikvah before you start trying to conceive. Traditional uses of mikvah deal with menstruation and pregnancy. Many Jewish women go each month to immerse themselves in the ritual bath after their period has ended. As you prepare physically to make a baby, visiting the mikvah can be a nice opportunity to prepare mentally and spiritually. It's a moment in time, separate from the hassle of daily routine, to really look inward and acknowledge the monumental change you and your body are about to experience. Going to the mikvah can be a good spiritual and ritualistic component to add to your routine, to help prepare your mind and heart for the next chapter of your life. Some women struggling with infertility may find going to the mikvah after their period or the loss of a pregnancy as a way to acknowledge each month as a new opportunity for getting pregnant, and a physical task to take part in at a time that otherwise can just be full of waiting.

One of the most helpful organizations when it comes to learning about the mikvah and finding one in your neighborhood that is welcoming is Mayyim Hayyim. Founder and President of the Board of Mayyim Hayyim, Anita Diamant, explained to me that the inspiration for creating the organization was to help make the mikvah accessible and welcoming to everyone in the Jewish community. She explained that immersing in the mikvah can be a way to honor the lifecycle events that women experience throughout their lives - from major ones like giving birth to smaller but still very poignant moments like when a mother's time nursing her baby comes to a close. Anita explained to me that the mikvah can offer a physical place to honor an experience that you want to ritualize. What's really wonderful about the Mayyim Hayyim associated mikvahs is that their policy is to never assume that someone has been to the mikvah before, so if you do decide to try it out and have any questions you will be able to find everything you need to know on the MayyimHayyim.com website.

The Jewish religion is very closely tied to many natural processes, and there are many ancient Jewish customs that actually show a profound knowledge of the human body and pregnancy. For example, the Gemara teaches us that we can pray for the gender of the baby up until the fortieth day after conception. In the Torah, Leah prayed for a girl during this time and gave birth to Dina. Biologically speaking, this is around the time (7 weeks) when a fetus begins to differentiate between male and female sex organs.

Rabbi Sara explained that the number 40 is often used in Jewish stories when referring to a "metamorphosis"—when things come to be—like the number of years the Jewish people wandered in the desert before reaching the promised land, during which time they received the Torah. Forty is also the number of days Moses spent on Mt. Sinai, where he received the Ten Commandments. And in Kabbalah, 40 also represents the four corners of our spiritual world which together make up the *sefirot*, also known as the elements of God. Each of the four corners is said to contain 10 *sefirot* (divine powers). In Hebrew, the number 40 is also denoted by the Hebrew letter *mem*. And the origin of the Hebrew letter *mem* is linked to the Hebrew word *mayim*, which means water—the universal source of life.

And 40 doesn't stop there. It is, of course, the number of weeks of a pregnancy. Rabbi Sara explained that there's a sense of this over-arching connection to human fertility throughout the Torah, in the "Jewish architecture of time." This connection resonates as we see the number 40 and other symbolic connections to the reproductive timeline popping up again and again.

The mitzvah of sex—let's get physical!

In Judaism, sex is a holy commandment—a mitzvah—and is considered the ultimate act of continuing God's work of creating the world. In traditional Jewish perspectives sex should be joyous; it's considered sinful to have sex only for one individual's pleasure to the exclusion of their partner. In the Torah the Hebrew word for sex is *yodeah*, which means "to know." Now that's a beautiful and powerful concept—when you are with your partner intimately, you may allow them to truly know you. The first commandment, or mitzvah, in the Torah is to procreate: God commands his people to "be fruitful and multiply" (Genesis 1:28). The word for the marriage ceremony is *kiddushin,* which comes from the Hebrew word *kadosh,* or "holy."

There's something special about making a baby that can be different from just general lovemaking. If you're actively trying to have a baby, you may be acutely aware of how important it is to treat your body well as a first step in creating a welcoming home for new life. Although the human body may always be ready for sex, Jewish law is concerned with preparing the mind for this physical experience. When a new life is created, Jewish people believe that God acted in part with man and woman to create it. We pray daily, *"Elohai nishma* - Oh God, the soul which you gave me is pure. You created it, you fashioned it, you breathed it into me."

Did you know it's a mitzvah to have sex? Judaism is all about the marriage of the physical and the spiritual. Enjoying life and finding pleasure within the physical world is part of Judaism. Your body and your sexuality are not sinful. Hooray!

Man and wife are encouraged to have sex on Shabbat, as this is considered a holy time and a moment when they take time to bless one another and their family; their mind and soul are in the right place for it. You may have heard the term "double mitzvah" used as a joke, but there's a lot of truth to the sentiment. Women are encouraged to immerse themselves in the mikvah (ritual bath, see more in Chapter 3) before each cycle as a way to spiritually prepare for sex, because it is regarded as a holy act.

If you're someone who is conceiving via in vitro fertilization (IVF), there are opportunities to talk to your partner about how the many difficult medical procedures could involve some elements of sacred connection you might miss, if that appeals to you.

The Torah and rabbis who teach Jewish law talk about the two mitzvot of *pru urvu* (procreation) and *onah* (marital intimacy). These are two separate things, and they each complement and heighten the other. Jewish teachings often mention elevating the physical world, and sex with your partner is one of the ultimate ways to do so. Judaism even protects a woman's right be satisfied sexually, even when she and her husband are not trying to get pregnant, or even if the couple is not able to conceive at all.

It is written in the Torah: " Hence a man leaves his father and mother and clings to his wife, so that they become one flesh." (Beresheet 2:24). The Hebrew word used here for cling is *davak*; Jewish scholars write about what this means, and how fulfilling and positive it is for two people to be joined so intimately. OK, enough about rabbis and sex...the point is, if you aren't enjoying a sexually satisfying relationship with your partner you should speak up. It's the Jewish thing to do.

Mayim Bialik wrote an article for Kveller.com called "Mayim Bialik Talks About Sex." In that article, she said, "Judaism loves love. We love sex. We are told it is a mitzvah to make love and to especially make love on Shabbat, when God's presence is close. A woman's right to sexual satisfaction is detailed in her ketubah, her marriage contract." Sex is not a forbidden, dangerous or evil event, it is a celebrated component of who we are as humans and Jews!

So as you go forth to participate in the act of creation, just re- member that however you and your partner go about it, we are all created *b'tzelem Elohim*—in the image of God—and our desires for love and sex are no exception. So consider yourself officially Jewishly blessed to make a baby!

Judaism's thoughts on sex don't all revolve around love and spir- ituality; in fact, the Torah is pretty prescriptive about how to go about procreating. It says to count for yourself seven days after your period has ended as a good time to start trying. Three thousand years later, science still says that a woman's most fertile days are generally around the twelfth day of her cycle. For centuries, this twelfth day has been the traditional day that Jewish women have immersed in the mikvah in preparation for getting pregnant.

You may be surprised to find out that Jewish law gets pretty specific when it comes to a woman's period and when she and her husband can have sex. A woman takes on a specific status when she is menstruating, called *niddah*; when her body has finished that cycle, the status changes to *tehorah* at which point she can immerse in the mikvah. Strictly observant women will not return to marital relations with their husbands until their period has ended; in fact it's forbidden! The time period of this separation is called *onat perishah*. Many Orthodox women feel that this forced separation can be a blessing in a marriage because it makes the return to one another that much sweeter. It also can serve as a time of self-care and self-reflection for a woman. As mentioned earlier, the timing of returning to the marital bed after a woman's period also matches that of a woman's most fertile days.

You've done the prep work (sex) and now it's time to take the test—the pregnancy test

So you've been trying and praying and hoping for that little extra line to pop up on a pregnancy test (or maybe you haven't); and the day finally arrives. Personally, I've taken a whole bunch of pregnancy tests; each experience was a terrifying three-minute ordeal of nervous anticipation. I am very guilty of testing too early in my cycle. But those dang tests are just so tempting sitting in their little packages, knowing so much more than you do, holding the ability to tell the future. The only thing that really stopped me from daily testing when I was trying for a baby was knowing that testing every day could get really expensive. The waiting game of pregnant or not pregnant is torture—as if the waiting game the rest of the nine months isn't!

Three minutes—that's the standard amount of time a lady needs to wait before the results are revealed. Unless, like me, you test too early and then you also need to spend 20 minutes frantically scouring the internet for pictures of 'faint lines' on positive tests.

If you've just taken a test for the first time, I want you to stop and take a moment to really commit to memory what the experience was like. It really is a rite of passage in this modern world, sort of like buying your first box of period products. It's a drug-store bequeathed threshold into a whole new life.

If you've gotten that double blue line, or plus sign, or PREG-NANT word on a pregnancy test (or perhaps all three because you just wanted to confirm it, again!) let me be the first to say 'B'shaah Tovah'! You are participating in a miracle. E

ach one of us is created in God's image—*b'tzelem Elohim*— so it's as though we have a piece of God and God's holiness within us. When we bring a child into this world we are adding more holiness, more Godliness to Earth.

2.

Pregnancy Loss & Pregnancy Termination

Why begin at the end? Well, if you're at this point and have reached the end of a pregnancy, I don't want to put you through the heartache of having to flip through the rest of this book to find what you're looking for. I also want to raise awareness that this happens; it happens more than we'll maybe ever know, and it helps to talk about it. Or, at least, it helped me to talk about it.

Judaic text and generations of rabbis hold deep sympathy and understanding for a woman who is struggling to bear a child. The story of Hannah in the Bible, who could not bear children for many years, is used as a cornerstone symbol in the Yom Kippur High Holiday service as the prime example of how someone should pray. Her whole physical being was so overcome with the experience of prayer, asking God for a child, that she was thought to be drunk. God saw her suffering and answered her prayers, gave her a son whom she named Samuel, and in turn she gave him to the Holy Temple to devote his life to God. It's a complex story with many layers of meaning, but I think the message that 'if you pray hard enough you will have a child' is not the true or most profound takeaway from Hannah's story. Instead, I highlight the story of Hannah here to show how ancient Jewish text acknowledges how deep the all-encompassing desire to have a child can be.

Here is how the Book of Samuel records Hannah's prayer:

> In her wretchedness, she prayed to God, weeping all the while.
>
> And she made this vow: "O Lord of Hosts, if You will look upon the suffering of Your maidservant and will remember me and not forget Your maidservant, and if You will grant Your maidservant a male child, I will dedicate

him to God for all the days of his life; and no razor shall ever touch his head."

Jewish tradition during pregnancy loss

Judaism is an ancient religion with much ritual originating in a time before the advent of modern medicine. As a result, Jewish practice around pregnancy—and pregnancy loss especially—can feel outdated. Pregnancy loss is such a core-striking event in a woman's life because it can shift your vision of who you are and who you want to be—a mother. While other life cycle events are centered in their religious observances (becoming an adult, getting married, etc.), there is no Jewish ritual for pregnancy loss.

Maharat Ruth Balinsky Friedman of Temple Ohev Shalom in Washington, D.C. is one of the first ordained female Orthodox rabbis. She explained to me that many Jewish women struggle with the fact that Judaism has no official support structure for them at this time. She counsels women who are looking for something to do—a prayer to say, a way to grieve—that fits into their spiritual practice.

The historical explanation for why Judaism doesn't acknowledge the loss of an unborn baby in the same way the secular world might is because the Jewish mourning rituals (three months of shiva, abstaining from daily life) are especially burdensome. Miscarriages and pregnancy losses happened so often hundreds of years ago that it was impractical to require women to honor them in the same way. But, it can feel isolating and unfair to someone who otherwise expects Judaism to be there for all of their major milestones.

Although there are not specific mourning rituals that Jewish people must observe for pregnancy loss, there are many Jewish sources for ritual and spiritual comfort during this hard time. Pregnancy loss can be an extremely isolating experience. Judaism can serve women at this heartbreaking time in their lives, and Jewish law can be a source of wisdom to lean on. Rabbi Shira Stutman of 6th and I expressed to me that Judaism offers a meaningful spiritual tradition for families during these times. Even for those who are not religious; who don't keep kosher—"Like a mountain, whether you choose to hike it or not," she explained to me, Jewish tradition is always there."

Finding community, reaching out

When I experienced pregnancy loss I felt tremendously alone, almost like an outcast, with a bad luck stigma hanging over me. I thought I brought sadness and awkward conversation to every room I entered, so I instinctively stayed home. When I did see friends I pretended: I wore a smile, I asked questions about their lives and made conversation so they didn't have to. I was tempted to look online for comfort; maybe a chat room? I know they are helpful for some people but I found them to be, well...depressing. Full of terribly sad stories, each one more tragic than the next. And while these support communities can be lifelines for thousands of women, it can really help to reach out beyond the screen.

I am a very shy person and didn't have the interest in this so I can only speak to what happened a few months after my experience with loss. I started to be on the receiving end of requests for comfort and support, and I was glad to be able to offer it. Once you're in this world, you're part of the secret society and a world opens up.

Rabbi Dara Frimmer of Temple Isaiah in West Los Angeles kindly shared with me her experience with stillbirth. She said, "Before I had a stillbirth I didn't know anyone that had one; then once I did I was flooded with people who had and wanted to talk about it." You might not realize it, but "the community is there." Rabbi Dara now finds that being willing to publicly share stories helps spread awareness and visibility, and contributes to this community of support. As a rabbi she finds special significance in the ways Judaism honors loved ones who have died and how much this resonates to her as an important part of our tradition.

Within the Jewish community on Instagram there is a hashtag #realloverealloss started by the amazing influencer Elizabeth Savetsky, where women share stories of their own experiences with pregnancy loss. In part this movement was started to end the stigma (especially in the more religious communities) surrounding miscuarriage and infertility and to show how common it sadly is. If you are facing infertility and looking for community, search the hashtag and consider reaching out to the women sharing their stories who post that they are open to connecting. Below is a poem by Lauren Sussman, who was just a friend of a friend to me but is now truly a friend of mine. We connected after she lost a pregnancy and helped each other to heal.

Secret Society
A poem by Lauren Sussman
We are survivors.
We are sisters.
We feel each other's pain.
Our hearts break for once and another.
We pick each other up.
We are part of a secret society.
One that no one wants to join.
But there is strength in knowing you are not alone.
As we pass by each other
We can see right through the masks
we wear.
We are the strongest and most compassionate people.
We are sensitive.
We share the same perspective.
We take one step at a time.
We stand still when everyone moves forward.
We repeat to ourselves that it's okay,
and we are okay.
And we are not okay.
Nothing about what happened to us is okay.

It is cruel!

It is pain.

It rips us open when we least expect it.

But it makes us stronger.

It teaches us to love harder.

It teaches us to be hopeful.

You give me hope sister.

Without you, I stand alone.

I am never alone, because of you,

Thank you sister.

Steps to heal after loss

While healing isn't a science, there are things you can to do try to heal your heart. I won't say that life will ever return to "normal" because I believe a life event like this profoundly changes a person and it can never be erased. And it shouldn't be; because however short the experience was, it's part of you and who you are.

My own story isn't the worst one I've heard (by far) but I think I've gained compassion for pregnancy stories that end before they're expected to. Since I lost my first pregnancy in 2015 I have spoken to many women suffering similar circumstances, and have become a sort of de-facto "can you walk me through this" advisor. Unfortunately many of these connections are made in hidden text message conversations, as women are still embarrassed and afraid to speak out about their suffering.

I reached out to Rabbi Shira Stutman of Sixth and I Synagogue in Washington, D.C. during my time of crisis, and she had many wise words for me. I told her to ask me to run a marathon; to make me do 1,000 push-ups; to assign me some painful, exhausting task I could accomplish that would somehow in turn alleviate my unbearable emotional pain. She told me, of course, that even if I did all that, the pain would still be there; that only time and emotional peace would heal the wounds. She advised me to go to the mikvah and create my own ceremony to say goodbye to all that I had lost.

Rabbi Stutman also shared some really unique advice. She told me I didn't have to tell anyone what exactly happened with my pregnancy. She explained that people often 'just want to know' as a sort of emotional check, an instinctive way for them to assess how you should feel and to see if they might be in danger of something similar happening to them. So as a way to protect my privacy, and to honor the pregnancy that I lost, I chose to never share exactly what happened. It's been one of the few things I've been allowed to control and I am forever grateful for that advice.

Saying goodbye

There is an unfortunate attitude of secrecy and guilt toward pregnancy loss that is only now dissipating in many Jewish communities. Many millennial women have grown up in a Jewish culture that celebrates feminine strength (we put an orange on the Seder plate; we pray at the Kotel; we engage in feminist discussions each month at Rosh Chodesh), but we don't discuss our periods with our rabbis, and we are still very private and discreet about pregnancy. The combination of superstition and modesty (also known as *shnius*) creates an atmosphere where these things are "just not talked about." As a result, Judaism can feel alienating, harsh and unwelcoming during struggles with infertility and pregnancy loss. But that's changing.

While it will take time for synagogues to evolve, it shouldn't stop you from reaching out to your rabbi or someone you trust within your own synagogue to let them know what's happened. There may be support groups or other resources within your local Jewish community. It can also be a time to speak to your rabbi about praying with them or asking for help to guide you toward prayers that would be especially helpful at this time.

Some families choose to have a burial of the remains after a pregnancy loss; others feel this would be too painful or inappropriate, depending on what they believe about what they lost. Though there is no formal Jewish ceremony or funeral for pregnancy loss, you can ask your rabbi to join you, say some words of prayer and offer a time for you to say goodbye.

Rabbi Danielle Eskow from OnlineJewishLearning.com experienced pregnancy loss in her own journey to motherhood and found the same lack of support within the Jewish community that many other women have experienced. There weren't obvious resources like prayers to say and rituals to observe. Jewish mourning rituals are extensive—full of meaning, prayer and physical expressions of grief, as well as reconnection to life. Rabbi Eskow sought her own way to incorporate the Jewish rituals that she observes during other significant life cycle events. She decided to go to the mikvah as one of the first concrete acts of healing. In a beautiful "full circle" moment, she went back to that mikvah in her 9th month of pregnancy with her first daughter.

Another helpful resource for spiritual understanding during dark days is Rabbi Harold Kushner's book *When Bad Things Happen to Good People*. This is one of the most popular modern Jewish books; it presents a way to relate to God and to make sense of how tragedy can occur to people who don't deserve it. He focuses the book on how to think of God and understand random circumstances in a way that can reaffirm your Judaism to provide comfort and support during a difficult time.

Personally I felt I needed to create a mourning ritual to say goodbye and begin to close this chapter of my life. There aren't any rules here of course, so I encourage you to think about what would feel meaningful to you. I didn't want to include anyone else in this ceremony besides myself and my husband, but I wanted us to do something to officially say goodbye to this pregnancy. We created two personal rituals. First, I read *Tears of Sorrow, Seeds of Hope* by Rabbi Nina Cardin, a book to help those dealing with infertility and pregnancy loss. In this book I found prayers that I wanted to include in our personal ritual. We chose a meaningful spot in a beautiful setting for the day. As much as I dreaded the ceremony, I also looked forward to this meaningful goodbye.

Here is a passage that I chose to use for my ceremony, excerpted from *Tears of Sorrow, Seeds of Hope* by Rabbi Nina Cardin.

> Oh God, I commend back to Your safekeeping the potential life entrusted to me for so short a time, even as I grieve its passing out of the protection of my body.
>
> You created the miracle of birth and the wonder of the body that cares for mother child. *Dayan Ha'emet*, Righteous Judge, You care for Your creatures even when such care tastes bitter. *Haracham*, Merciful One, heal my body and soul, that I may come to sing Your praises as a happy mother surrounded by her children in the courtyards of a Jerusalem at peace.
>
> God heals the broken-hearted.
> And binds their wounds.
> God reckons the number of stars,
> Giving each one its name.
> Great is God and full of power
> Whose wisdom is beyond reckoning
> God gives courage to the lowly
> And brings hope to those bereft.
> So may God always be with us.
> —based on Psalm 147:2-6

The second thing that we did was pray together with our rabbi, just the three of us, in front of the *aron kodesh* (the ark which holds the Torah scrolls in synagogue). Our rabbi, Rabbi Weinblatt of Congregation B'nai Tzedek, took us into the synagogue after speaking to him about what we had experienced and we prayed. Just knowing that someone else dedicated a few minutes to pray for our healing and future blessings was a powerful moment of hope.

It can also be extremely helpful and necessary to talk to a therapist. I made the mistake of not doing this soon enough!

Setting a time to mourn

In Judaism, when someone dies, it's customary to mourn him or her for a specific time period. I think this concept of designating time to mourn isn't so much about making sure people's memories are properly honored, although that's a nice benefit. The greater blessing of this tradition is that it specifies the mourners' grieving time. And when it's not time to mourn, it's time to live again— to embrace the light and love of the world as it is and not dwell in the world to come.

There are no Jewish customs when it comes to pregnancy loss; in fact, there's no halachic burial ritual for a child who dies before their first birthday. These laws were, of course, written when infant mortality was extremely high. In today's world it's shocking to think that a newborn wouldn't receive a funeral if he or she passed away. But where Judaism is really lacking is in how it addresses pregnancy loss. Because a baby is not considered to be alive until it's born (or more strictly speaking, halfway out of its mother), there are no mourning protocols for neonatal loss.

When I lost a baby at five months pregnant, I spent a lot of time researching this, seeking rabbis' counsel and ultimately creating my own spiritual mourning ritual. The first thing I did was set aside a specific mourning period—three months. This is a traditional time period in Judaism; when someone dies, their immediate relatives observe shiva for three months. In this time they refrain from attending parties or celebrations, and they say the kaddish prayer.

This was a helpful decision for me. It allowed me to observe my own mourning time. Most importantly, it helped define an end to the mourning period. I wasn't sure if I would ever feel right going to parties and being social again, but when those three months ended, I forced myself to give it a try, and slowly it became normal again.

Designating a mourning period gave me structure, meaning, and normalcy in this difficult time in my life.

I also think it's helpful to set a time during the day to mourn. For me it was while driving to and from work and during my lunch break, when I would take a walk. That basically resulted in a few chunks of time where I didn't cry or break down because I knew I would have that designated time later in the day. But I also had an emergency backup. If I couldn't make it to the next block of time, I would write out how I was feeling (usually with good old fashioned pen and paper). This small physical element gave me a release and allowed me to focus and get my thoughts out. During my "crying times" in the car, I put on my "sad times" playlist and just let it all out. I cranked up the volume and cried my heart out. Twenty minutes later, when I arrived at work or back home, I felt exhausted and empty, but not panicked—not on the edge of sadness. I embraced the sadness, fully, and then was ready to return to some level of normalcy for the rest of the day.

Jewish prayer can be a helpful source of comfort during this painful time. Just as songs will likely take on new meaning as you relate quotes and phrases to your personal experience, so can prayer take on a higher spiritual power. It can also be a roller coaster, and that's OK. Some days prayer will be meaningless, painful and strange. Other times a familiar refrain will pull you to tears. That's OK, too. It doesn't hurt to try it and find out if helps you. I grew up trained in prayer—we prayed every day in school. So for me it was a familiar task to help me focus my attention and do something. Some days I didn't pray to God; I just enjoyed the melodies and the moment to sit in my own thoughts, undistracted, as a form of meditation.

Finally, when the mourning period that I had set aside (three months) had concluded, I visited the mikvah—the Jewish ritual bath. From that experience I learned that the mikvah is an amazing resource for women to create an extremely personal and resonating ritual. Immersing in the ritual bath—being completely enclosed in water—can be a physical and emotional rebirth. The organization Mayyim Hayyim has rituals and resources available on their website MayyimHayyim.org where you can find a specific miscarriage and pregnancy ceremony to use when you visit the mikvah.

I found that choosing something to signify an end to the mourning period, like going to the mikvah—although it could be reading a special poem, saying a prayer or just going on a walk to a meaningful place—can really help. In Rabbi Cardin's book, she also proposes the idea of using *Havdalah* as a way to say goodbye. As *Havdalah* means "separation," it is a natural moment of separating between two things. Each week it is used to mark the separation of Shabbat from the rest of the week; but you might find it meaningful to define a separation between a time period of grief and one of renewal and healing. Having this formal type of ending can allow you to give yourself permission to begin to think about the future and begin to turn part of your heart to life once again.

Terminating a pregnancy

One highly politicized arena where religion and pregnancy meet is in the ethics of abortion. A Pew Religious Landscape Survey in 2007 found that 84% percent of American Jews support legalized abortion in all or most cases, and most Rabbis and Jewish communities support a women and her right to choose. The historical reasoning behind this divergence of thought between Judaism and many other religions is that Judaism does not consider a fetus to be a life of its own until it is halfway out of the mother. It is for this reason that abortion has been allowed if, for example, the pregnancy is putting the mother's life in danger. Today many Jewish thinkers have expanded this message of compassion to the fetus and with genetic testing and advanced early ultrasounds also allow for abortions when the child would be born into a life of suffering and pain.

If you are faced with this impossible choice in your pregnancy there is a good (albeit very emotional) book on the topic called

Our Heartbreaking Choices by Christie Books, a collection of short stories of women sharing their experiences choosing to terminate a pregnancy due to medical complications.

American Jews tend to lean more toward pro-choice on the political scale, especially in progressive communities that embrace a woman's right to determine what happens to her body. Rabbi Stutman explained to me that because in Judaism a baby is not considered alive until it's born, especially at the beginning, the fetus is just another part of the gestational carrier's body,

There's an old Jewish story about the famous Rabbi Judah Hanasi, who edited the Mishnah text. He was a wise and celebrated teacher; as he aged, his following of young and fervent disciples grew. As he neared the end of his life, his health waned and his students came to his home to pray for him around the clock. Their constant urgency begging God not to take him made it so that he couldn't pass into the world to come. One of his handmaidens saw his suffering and knew it was wrong. So, she smashed a piece of pottery on the ground so that it made a loud crashing noise. For a moment there was silence as everyone turned to see what had happened. In this moment Judah Hanasi was allowed to die. This story is used throughout Jewish ethical discussion to support the idea of compassionate care, hospice and medically assisted suicide.

A woman who chooses to become pregnant and is then forced to terminate a pregnancy due either to the medical danger to herself or the fetus for continuing is often left bereft and angry after the experience. To Jewish women in this situation I recommend the same mourning rituals and steps to healing described earlier in this chapter. With this experience, as with other pregnancy loss, there can be a lot of challenges to your faith and anger at God. There's no easy answer to this but it's an extra scar that can last after the baby is gone. Finding healing through counseling and mourning can help you return to a faith in God or spirituality that can once again be a source of comfort to you.

Stillbirth and third trimester loss

A loss at any stage of pregnancy can have a profound effect on a woman and on a family. There is no *rule of weeks*: that a loss at 20 weeks is 10 times harder than a loss at 10 weeks etc. However, the women I spoke with who had lost babies in the third trimester or who had experienced a stillbirth often experienced the loss in a way that is comparable to the loss of a child. Many took part in formal burials or had the chance to see or hold their babies before saying goodbye. If you have suffered this type of loss or have received news from your doctor that it is likely, I encourage you to talk to a rabbi and/or mental health professional about working together through grief counseling or to create a ceremony to say goodbye.

Stillbirth and neonatal loss can be devastating for a family. We know that miscarriage is common during the first few weeks of pregnancy—so much so that people often don't share news that they're expecting until this stage has passed. However, once this delicate time has passed many women treat the rest of their pregnancy as a given – get through the next few months and a healthy baby will arrive. Medical knowledge and the use of ultrasounds are so advanced now that it is truly shocking when there is an instance of neonatal death.

Traditionally, Jewish law does not consider a baby to have lived if they do not reach 30 days of life. This 30-day mark is when the rabbis considered the baby's life to be viable. In his MyJewishLearning.com essay entitled 'How to Mourn Stillbirth and Neonatal Death' Dr. Ron Wolfson, a preeminent leader in the Jewish community and Fingerhut Professor of Education at American Jewish University in Los Angeles, explains that this custom is based on these two Jewish sources:

> "We do not mourn for fetuses *(nefalim)*, and anything
> which does not live for 30 days, we do not mourn for it."
> — Maimonides, *Mishneh Torah*, Hilkhot Aveilut 1:6

"The infant, for 30 days, even including the full 30th day (if it dies), we do not mourn for it"
— Yoseph Karo, *Shulchan Aruch*, Yoreh De-ah 374:8

In the past few decades Jewish rituals surrounding loss in the third trimester and stillbirth have changed. It is customary to revisit how we interpret Jewish law with each generation and the Conservative movement established new laws in the 1990s on how a baby lost late in pregnancy or a stillborn baby should be buried and mourned. This change was influenced in large part by how the especially painful and tragic experience of these types of losses are felt today.

Dr. Ron Wolfson explains: "The tremendous sense of loss and the overwhelming need to grieve felt by the parents of an infant who dies before the thirty-day benchmark does not go away just because the *halacha* prevents the mourning rituals from taking place."

Today many psychologists advise couples to see and touch their babies before they are buried, to take photos of them and with them, and to safely store keepsakes from those precious few days.

Rabbi Stephanie Dickstein wrote in a paper approved by the Committee of Jewish Law and Standards of the Rabbinical Assembly, which provides guidance on halachah for the Conservative community, that the need for a change in Jewish law is based on three tenets. First, that there is a strong and very real emotional connection to a stillborn baby. Second, that *potential* life exists in this situation—which means there is a level of holiness and respect that it deserves. And third, improved medical technology today has resulted in the expectation that a baby born during the third trimester will live.

The Conservative movement adopted the recommendation based on Rabbi Dickstein's work that when the mother has recovered physically from the experience, she should recite the *Birkat HaGomel* which is used when someone has survived a dangerous situation like a surgery or car accident. In response, the community should visit the mother and family and observe the mitzvah of *bikur cho-lim*—visiting the sick.

The funeral and burial at a Jewish cemetery for a stillborn baby should be held as soon as possible but not before the mother is able to attend. The baby should be given a Hebrew name and *kaddish* (the traditional Jewish mourning prayer) recited for them, and the family should sit shiva and observe mourning rituals.

This change in Jewish law by the Conservative movement also very specifically states that the adoption of these mourning rituals should in no way raise concern over the permissibility of abortion. A late-term abortion is permissible if the pregnancy is causing a serious threat to the mother's health or the fetus has been diagnosed with a condition that would seriously affect it.

What to know, what to say

Jewish spiritual teachings say that we live in a shattered, broken world. When we break the glass on our wedding day part of the symbolism of this exuberant act is to remind us of that very fact. It is our job as agents of God to spend our lives doing our best to repair what is broken in the world; this is the notion of *tikkun olam*. Judaism teaches that there are three ways to repair the world—three elements of human behavior that are essential to living a holy life. In the Talmud it says that the entire world rests on these three pillars: "*Torah, avodah* (work) and *gemilut hasadim* (acts of righteousness)"—Pirkei Avot 1:2. Visiting the sick, comforting those who are mourning and those who are facing personal struggles are among the highest form of *mitzvot* in Judaism. If someone you know is facing a broken, difficult time in their life—which pregnancy loss most definitely is—it is a core aspect of Judaism to support them.

Jewish Philosopher Emanuel Levinas teaches that meaning in life comes from our ability to respond to this brokenness in the world. He believed that there is meaning within suffering because it provides the impetus for others to help. People respond when someone is suffering, and that brings God into our world. By helping others, we fulfill a divine aspect of being human, therefore suffering provides this opening for God in our lives. It is not "Jewish" to ignore a tragedy like this; it is Jewish to respond with kindness and support.

When my husband and I found out we were going to be losing our pregnancy, I remember saying to him that he should probably email our friends and family. I figured that was the best way of distributing the news so that I didn't have to have the same awkward, depressing conversation over and over again. I figured there might actually be some nice email responses to read later that week, and that thought was comforting to me. When we returned home from the hospital after experiencing our loss, one of the first things I did was call my closest friend; I just said, "Come over." This is very, very unlike me; I usually have so much social anxiety and am not one of those girls who's always going here and there with girlfriends for coffees or mani/pedis. I just arrived home and was instantly compelled to be with people. She and her husband sat (literally) at my bedside and we just chatted. I don't know how else I would have survived the afternoon. By the next day our home was full of flowers, cards, meals and treats from friends, colleagues and family.

I have never in my life felt as supported and cared for. Those gifts were emotionally worth 10 times what we received when we got married or when my son was born. Each one felt like a totally unexpected surprise and I still remember and truly appreciate them all to this day. Even more, I remember the people who checked in—even weeks and months later—to see how I was doing. In my personal experience those who had experienced their own loss (not necessarily a pregnancy, but maybe a parent or other similarly heartbreaking event) knew that reaching out was helpful. A lot of people think that not bringing it up is more helpful, or they can be shy and uncomfortable when they first see you; I totally understand that. From my experience and the women I interviewed, t even just the shortest text message and check-in is helpful.

There is a Jewish organization called NechamaComfort which offers a downloadable guide on their website (*nechamacomfort.com*) to help and comfort those suffering pregnancy loss and infant loss. The organization is dedicated to helping all family members, including extended family deal with the loss.

I asked Dalia Davis, the President of *Uprooted: A Jewish Response to Fertility Journeys*, if there were any misunderstandings about Judaism and pregnancy loss that she felt were important to clear up. These are the *Big Three*:

1. People don't know how common this is. There's a recurring theme that Dalia pointed out that I also noticed when interviewing women for this book, almost everyone who experienced pregnancy loss felt like they were 'the only one' they knew who was suffering through this. The tendency to keep the loss experience private has resulted in a lack of support and community because when someone does go through this they don't realize that there are so many others in similar situations they could be reaching out to.

2. Some Jewish women are told that if they pray hard enough they will have a child. This advice isn't always intended to misdirect or psychologically harm a woman who has experienced pregnancy loss, but hearing this type of rhetoric can create a false sense of control and self-blame during these events which can be damaging psychologically. It also can distort a woman's perception of faith and God when her prayers, however devout, aren't answered.

3. Along the same lines the phrase "I'll pray for you" is another form of victim blaming that often isn't comforting to a woman who has experienced a loss. Although it's again intended with love and concern, the logic behind the statement can twist into the same notion that if only the mother had prayed hard enough, she wouldn't be facing this reality.

When I talk about how to help someone heal I just keep two rules of compassion in mind, which I believe are helpful rules for oneself and for others. 1: Never dismiss the pain. 2: Never offer platitudes. One person's experience with a loss in the first weeks of pregnancy can feel as painful to them as someone else's loss in the third trimester. It's impossible to compare suffering and it also isn't helpful to hear "It could always be worse." My second rule is to avoid phrases like "everything happens for a reason" and "you'll have another baby soon" firstly, because I find these sentiments illogical and untrue; and second, because when a woman has just lost a pregnancy it isn't necessarily comforting to hear that this loss shouldn't hurt so much because they will likely have a healthy child in the future. They are not interchangeable and one doesn't negate the pain of the other. I also encourage anyone suffering from grief to reach out, reach out to friends, reach out to a therapist, just don't hide and suffer alone.

3.

Infertility

What's Jewish about infertility? Unfortunately, a lot.

There's a lot of pressure within Jewish religious tradition and Jewish culture to "be fruitful and multiply." So what does that mean when you're a "good" Jewish person who struggles to have a child? Although there's an impression from looking at Jewish religious communities where women seem to always have their arms full of children—that Jewish women easily have lots of kids—the facts, unfortunately, tell a very different story. According to statistics compiled by the Jewish Fertility Foundation, all three denominations in the Jewish community—which include the Reform, Conservative, and Orthodox movements—all equally experience decline in fertility due to maternal age.

The Jewish Fertility Foundation says Jewish women under the age of 30 suffer infertility at a rate of 1 in 10. Between the ages of 30-34, that number increases to 1 in 8; and between 35-36 it is as high as 1 in 6. With many couples trying for children later in life, the Jewish average infertility numbers are closer to 1 in 6 compared to the American national average of 1 in 8. So infertility can be a very Jewish journey.

The story of infertility within the Jewish community is not a new one. In fact, it is one of our most ancient narratives, beginning with the very first Jewish woman in the Torah—Abraham's wife Sarah. It wasn't until the age of 90 that Sarah was visited by the three strangers and was told she would have a child. Numbers can be a bit odd in the Bible, but the point here is that she had been waiting many years for this! Naturally, after years of deep sorrow at her inability to have a child, she laughed at the unexpected news.

Rabbi Stutman explained to me that Judaism is an "emotional

religion," and the tropes of women who were unable to bear children are woven throughout the Torah. Fertility struggles are at the forefront of the Rosh Hashanah service when we read about Hannah's inability to have a child.

Every year on the High Holidays the entire Jewish people, in every synagogue around the world, from the great Orthodox Schul in Jerusalem to the intimate gathering on the beach in Malibu, read the same story of Hannah's infertility. The Haftorah parshah centers on the figure of Hannah and her prayers to God through her struggle to have children. Her example is used as the epitome of what true devout prayer is. In the Biblical story Hannah's prayers are remembered by God and she does go on to have a child, Samuel whom she gives back to God as a servant at the Holy Temple. The idea of infertility and prayer is so closely tied to the Jewish High Holidays that the very first line of the Torah portion for the day begins by telling us that God remembered Sarah who was unable to have a child. The readings continue by looking at Rachel and Hannah and how they also struggled to conceive.

Dalia Davis, the President of *Uprooted: A Jewish Response to Fertility Journeys* explained to me that the Torah uses the prayers of the matriarchs asking God for a child as the ultimate example of what true and full prayer is. It is not a man following every letter of the law or reciting every word of a prayer book, it's a woman begging and bargaining with God for the ability to conceive and bring a healthy baby into this world. Infertility is part of our history and a defining element of Judaism. It cannot be explicated from who we are as a people and it is right there at the forefront of our story. If it is part of your story now, you are not alone.

Judaism holds children in extremely high regard, to have one is the ultimate mitzvah, and this is the counterpoint to infertility. Possibly it is because of these difficult lessons our ancestors experienced that we do treasure children as such precious blessings. They are the counterpoint to this shared struggle and so when one has a child in the Jewish faith they are celebrated from the moment they enter this world.

The Synagogue can be a lonely place

Have you ever heard the expression that some people feel most alone when they're surrounded by others? For someone experiencing infertility, a Jewish synagogue can really bring out that strange sensation. Synagogue life in Judaism revolves around the family. There are often activities for people of every age, but the two most prominent and active groups are usually the older generation of retirees who have time to devote the Sisterhood or volunteering, and the young families who attend the Tot Shabbats and send their children to the nursery school. American synagogues have a noticeably absent community of young couples who haven't yet had children. For a couple who have been trying to conceive, the synagogue unfortunately doesn't always often offer a community of support or even a spiritual place for hope and healing. Insensitive comments like, "When are you going to finally have a baby?" and "You should make your parents grandparents!" from well-meaning synagogue members make it worse. There are also couples who are experiencing secondary infertility, after having a first child but unable to conceive another. Comments like "when are you going to give so-and-so a baby sibling" can be very triggering. It hurts.

As prominent as the stories of childless matriarchs remain each year for Jews on the holiest days of the year, the infertility struggles for Jewish women today are not openly discussed much in the synagogue. Women suffering this wanting and longing aren't at the front and center of our daily prayers. Each time we pray we ask God in the Amidah to heal those who are sick—*refuah shleymah*—and each day we say Kaddish for those who have passed away. In each prayer service in synagogue there are so many specific things we as a community mention and openly pray for—but we don't hear about infertility or pregnancy loss. It's not mentioned in the Amidah or any of the central prayers of our everyday ritual readings, even though it features so prominently in the Torah. What are we to make of this dichotomy? For generations, many women have felt a sense of shame and secrecy and didn't speak openly in their Jewish communities about their experiences; but that is changing.

In an article by Maharat Ruth Friedman in the *Washington Post*, entitled "When you're facing infertility, a synagogue can be the most painful place to go. Let's change that," she shares how her personal journey of multiple miscarriages was a long and aching process. The synagogue for Ruth was a place where each celebration of a new baby stirred painful emotions of her own deep wanting. To inspire a message of change she wrote that communities need to be inclusive of everyone—those who are single or married; those who have children or who do not. And that during times of celebration synagogues also need to remember those who are suffering and make room for their pain with extra steps to welcome and engage them. Through articles like Friedman's we are slowly seeing a change in this generation as more Jewish networks of support become available to couples.

Gila Muskin Block is the founder Yesh Tikvah, a Jewish support organization for infertility. She explained to me that it is OK, and sometimes necessary, to take a step back and focus on your own self-care. Sometimes that means skipping synagogue events that are focused on family life, or avoiding walking by the line of strollers at the front door. These moments can be very triggering when you have such a strong desire to have a child of your own child be part of the community. Sometimes the answer is to give yourself space, feel your emotions, and work though them rather than deny them. Gila makes it very clear that while it is important to provide women with their own self determination to decide what they want to do, it's never OK to exclude women who you think may not want to attend such events.

The spiritual side effects of infertility as a Jewish woman

If you're struggling on a long and difficult infertility journey, you've likely experienced a range of emotions and reactions. Some women look toward Judaism and think, "What does this religion offer me now?" The synagogue is typically full of life celebrations: new babies being born; the simchas of bar and bat mitzvahs; children running up and down the hallways. This can be a triggering setting for a couple who is desperate for a child of their own. At this sensitive time women can feel like there's no place for them within the traditional synagogue community and may move away from their Judaism.

It's also especially common to feel stuck in a moment of spiritual disconnection. Where is God? Why is such a terrible thing happening to me when I have been a good person? When I have prayed? The idea of God can equally be a source of comfort or distress during this time.

In the Talmud it is said that there are three keys that only God can control: rain, bringing a soul back to life, and fertility. The rabbis teach that fertility therefore takes *more* than two people to make a baby (it turns out your eighth-grade sex-ed teacher was wrong!); God plays a role as well. Whether you believe in God or not, if you've struggled with pregnancy loss or infertility you have probably felt the acute unfairness of chance, fate or divine intervention however you want to understand it.

If you are in the midst of this very personal and spiritual struggle, know that feeling a visceral unfairness and anger at God can be very normal. Many of the women I spoke with felt guilt at their inability to continue to pray when their chances of conceiving seemed to be dwindling. Others expressed how their faith and prayer were sources of comfort during a long struggle.

And yet, when women eventually do become pregnant through medical intervention or otherwise, they tend to return to their equilibrium of faith and thank God for the gift of life they're now holding. One mother sent me her story to share her experience:

"We did struggle a bit," says Erin. "After some testing of both my husband and me, we found the issue seemed to be on his end and without medical interventions we weren't going to have a chance. He had just a scheduled an appointment with a specialist when we found out we miraculously were expecting. I definitely felt like there was a bit of divine intervention."

If you are someone who is struggling to understand the *why* in all of this, it may be helpful to speak to your rabbi or a support network; I'll share some resources in the next section. Suffering alone can make the suffering worse; the spiritual and emotional suffering that comes with infertility can be devastating.

Jewish resources for fertility journeys

Uprooted is an amazing Jewish organization dedicated to helping women heal during difficult pregnancies and struggles with infertility. I spoke with Dalia Davis, the president of Uprooted, who shared with me the impact her group is making in this area. The organization was born from the idea that someone can feel "uprooted" from who they are—their community and their vision of the future—when they struggle with building a family. Dalia explained that the organization was founded because there are so many amazing resources in the secular world for infertility struggles, but far fewer in the Jewish world.

Although infertility is so common in the Jewish population, Jewish couples often have to look outside their Jewish communities for the support they need. Uprooted can be a great resource for you if you're looking for a Jewish connection during this difficult life experience. They have a wide-reaching support network of mentors—other Jewish women and social workers from various backgrounds and in many locations across the United States who have had similar experiences and are available to talk. Uprooted is a safe space; unlike many secular infertility resources that try to sell their products or resources, Uprooted doesn't operate that way.

If you're reading this chapter you may be looking for a way to feel close to God again after a tragedy. Now, there are also places like Mayyim Hayyim who operate a network of mikvahs across the United States and provide a place to go for full support and healing. I spoke to author and Mayyim Hayyim founder and Board President Anita Diamant who shared with me that the organization was created as a community built project. Inspired by the idea of sharing the beauty and healing nature of mikvah with a wider audience, Mayyim Hayyim makes this ancient ritual accessible to the entire Jewish community. Part of what makes mikvahs associated with Mayyim Hayyim so welcoming is that they provide materials like prayer sheets with contemporary language and simple instructions and explanations for women looking for hope and healing during infertility journeys. I also personally recommend what is likely the most published Jewish book on the topic of grappling with God during difficult times—*When Bad Things Happen to Good People*, by Rabbi Harold Kushner.

The Yesh Tikvah organization has also been instrumental in contributing prayers and rituals for the Jewish community so that synagogues can be more welcoming to couples at this time of their life. They have instituted a custom on the holiday of Simchat Torah, the day we celebrate finishing reading the Torah and begin again, to include a Fertility Prayer.

Simchat Torah is a time when the synagogue is usually teeming with life as young children dance and sing and are celebrated. Even amidst all the celebration as we begin a new cycle of life for the Torah, this is an important time to remember those struggling to grow their own families and, as Gila put it, to "include them in our hearts."

Sharing in this one prayer and creating ritual regarding the infertility experience can be healing and comforting. The prayer can be said during the *Kol Hanearim* aliyah to the Torah. Traditionally children are called up during this Torah reading and blessed under a huge tallis. The tradition stems from a desire to bless and protect those most vulnerable in our community. This is why this time is also ideal to remember couples facing infertility. If your synagogue does not include this custom you can mention it to your rabbi as they may not have heard of it.

Here is Yesh Tikva's Fertility Prayer, reprinted with permission.

יְהִי רָצוֹן מִלְּפָנֶיךָ ה' אֱ-לֹהֵינוּ וַא-לֹהֵי אֲבוֹתֵינוּ, שׁוֹמֵעַ תְּפִלָּה, שְׁמַע תְּפִלָּתֵנוּ, וּבָרֵךְ אֶת כָּל חֲשׂוּכֵי הַיְלָדִים. פָּקְדֵם לְטוֹבָה, וְיוֹלִידוּ בְּרַחֲמֶיךָ בָּנִים וּבָנוֹת, זַרְעָא חַיָּא וְקַיָּמָא.

עַיִן נוֹשְׂאִים הֵם לְךָ לַשָּׁמַיִם, לֵב שׁוֹפְכִים נִכְחֲךָ כַּמַּיִם. חַזְּקֵם וְאַמְּצֵם, וְגָמְלֵם חֲסָדִים טוֹבִים, וּשְׁלַח לָהֶם רְפוּאָה שְׁלֵמָה וְתֵן לָהֶם שַׁלְוַת הַנֶּפֶשׁ.

וּכְשֵׁם שֶׁפָּקַדְתָּ אֶת שָׂרָה, רִבְקָה, רָחֵל וְחַנָּה, וְשָׁמַעְתָּ לְקוֹל הַצַּדִּיקִים וְהַצִּדְקָנִיּוֹת בְּשַׁוְּעָם אֵלֶיךָ, כֵּן תִּשְׁמַע לְקוֹל תְּחִנָּתֵנוּ. מַלֵּא מִשְׁאֲלוֹתֵינוּ לְטוֹבָה, וְקַבֵּל בְּרַחֲמִים וּבְרָצוֹן אֶת תְּפִלָּתֵנוּ. וְכֵן יְהִי רָצוֹן, וְנֹאמַר אָמֵן.

May it be Your will God, our Lord and the Lord of our forefathers, who answers prayers, hear our prayers and bless all those who struggle to have children. Remember them for good and with Your mercy they shall have sons and daughters, and grant them enduring offspring.

They lift up their eyes to You in heaven, they pour forth their hearts before You as water. Strengthen them and give them courage, grant them abundant kindness, heal them and help them find peace.

As you remembered Sarah, Rebecca, Rachel and Hannah, and You have heard the voices of the righteous men and women when they beseeched You, so too please listen to our outcry (to help the men and women of our community). Fulfill our wishes for good and accept with Your mercy and desire our prayers. And so may it be Your will, and let us say Amen.

The Yesh Tikvah organization also offers a multitude of other support options for couples to provide a Jewish response to the emotional and educational needs of couples. For example, they have a nationwide program called Fertility Friends which pairs two individuals on a similar journey—a mentor and mentee—to support one another. They also offer virtual support groups which are open to people all around the United States. The support groups are not just for the couples, but also for their parents and other extended family members affected. The Yesh Tikvah organization also has recorded lectures on infertility topics from medical doctors and mental health professionals. One other important awareness effort from Yesh Tikvah is the Infertility Awareness Shabbat program. This is an opportunity for extended family members to come together to share their experience of loss.

Another very helpful organization that you may want to touch base with is the Jewish Fertility Foundation. The Jewish Fertility Foundation is a partnership between the Jewish and medical community in the Southeast and is inclusive of all religious denominations as well as interfaith couples and everyone in between! One of the key services the organization offers is financial grants and loans for couples to pursue fertility treatments. They also offer private support groups online through Facebook, traditional in-person support groups, and a fertility buddies program to match "veterans" with "newbies." Please find a list of support organizations in the Resources section at the end of this book.

So, what to do?

The infertility experience can be a marathon of waiting and mental endurance. Sometimes there's nothing to do in between all the doctor appointments and test results. Here are some Jewish related activities that may be helpful to you:

❏ **Talk to your rabbi.**

You may be hesitant to share personal struggle with your rabbi, especially when it involves your body, and dare I say...sex! But you might be surprised to know that rabbis are, first of all, just people, and also are specially trained to help their congregants through crisis points in their lives. Chances are they have counseled many couples who have similar stories and will have words of comfort and a kind open heart for listening. You can also ask your rabbi to pray with you or to pray for you. While rabbis have no special direct line to God that you don't also have access to, it can feel especially comforting to know that someone else is joining you in your divine conversation and also praying on your behalf. If you don't belong to a synagogue you can still call or email a synagogue near you and ask to speak to a rabbi. It is customary in these circumstances to make a donation (of whatever amount feels comfortable to you, or you can ask the assistant if there is a recommended amount) as a thank you for the rabbi's time.

❏ **Read.**

In addition to the book by Dalia Davis, *Fertility Journeys: A Jewish Healing Guide* mentioned earlier, there is also a wealth of anecdotes and interviews with Jewish couples who struggled with infertility on the Jewish Fertility Foundation's website, www.jewishfertilityfoundation.org. These can be comforting and interesting, especially if you are feeling isolated in your experience. There are also many unique perspectives there so you may be able to read more about a specific condition that affects you. Other popular books that were recommended to me by the women I interviewed are:

Tears of Sorrow Seed of Hope: A Jewish Spiritual Companion for Infertility and Pregnancy Loss by Rabbi Nina Beth Cardin, and *Sh'ma, Be fruitful & multiply: A Jewish lens on infertility* by Naomi Less and Robyn Fryer Bodzin

❏ **Or Listen!**

Podcasts are another super helpful resource that was recommended time and time again by the women I interviewed for this book. Podcasts are convenient to listen to, have more varied perspectives, and can be more up-to-date than what's out in print. Here are some great ones:

Matt and Doree's Eggcellent Adventure. Doree is Jewish and a former Buzzfeed contributor, and Matt writes for *The Goldbergs* TV show. They began by podcasting their IVF journey and subsequent pregnancy and also include relatable stories from listeners who email in their personal experiences and questions.

IVFML. This is a miniseries sharing factual information from doctors and informed professionals led by Anna Almendrala, a senior editor at *HuffPost*, and her husband Simon Ganz.

❏ **Find Support.**

As mentioned in the section on Jewish resources for infertility, finding a supportive community can help you cope with the challenges of infertility. Though you may have the desire to turn inwards, and at times that is necessary and soothing, there are also times to push yourself to connect with others either through a counselor, a support group, or a friend who knows the intimate struggle you're facing.

❏ **Visit the Mikvah.**

Immersing in the mikvah in the hopes of getting pregnant is an ancient custom. There's an element of "good luck" that's spiritually tied to the experience and it's considered especially lucky to immerse after someone who is already pregnant.

Andria Kaplan, who writes the *ThatJewishWife* blog (www.thatjewishwife.com), told me that for two years through struggling to get pregnant, she became unable to go back to the mikvah because it was so closely associated with pregnancy; each month when she got her period again her heart was broken. After a hiatus she finally went back—not in the hope of becoming pregnant—just as a spiritual journey for herself, channeling an ancient ritual to reinvigorate her feminine personal power.

Andria's story had a happy ending and she did become pregnant after that immersion. But in her blog post about her mikvah experience (which she wrote before finding out she was pregnant), her message to her readers was to use the mikvah for personal reflection and empowerment when the focus of wanting to be pregnant becomes too much.

What NOT to say!

After interviewing many women who had experienced this type of struggle, I asked each of them what things people said to them that were meant to be helpful but actually really hurt. Here is their list. Some of these comments were directed at people who experienced secondary infertility—where the family had already given birth to one child but desired another; or after a miscarriage:

"Just relax. Go on vacation."

"You just need to not be so stressed out."

"At least you know you can get pregnant."

"At least you weren't too far along."

"God has a plan."

"Everything happens for a reason."

"Well you already have a child / career!"

"It's just not your turn."

"You just need to pray."

"I know so-and-so and she did such-and-such and she had a baby."

Expecting Jewish!

The First Trimester

4.

Nurturing the Mama:
Morning Sickness & Exhaustion

There's a new appreciation of an ancient Jewish value: *treat yo' self*! Self-love and self-care are core components of Judaism. After all, we are all created in the image of God—*b'tzelem Elohim*. So to love God is to love ourselves. And of course, if we are going to perform an ultimate (maybe **the** ultimate) act of creation by giving birth, then we need to care for ourselves first. *#Selfcare* may seem like an overused millennial hashtag these days, but I was amazed to hear how many women put themselves last—even when their body is working overtime to make a baby.

Women can stress out *so much* about owning the perfect items to care for and protect their babies: from organic cotton onesies to come home from the hospital in, to the safest car seat available on the market. Sometimes, however, we forget that our baby is already bundled up in the best baby carrier around: the womb! The effect of stress, diet, dehydration and exhaustion can all affect life in the womb.

As Jews we've been told to rest, relax, and take care of ourselves since the beginning: it's called Shabbat! A divinely ordained order to take a break from all the stress and stimulation of life and just *be*. Shabbat can be a beautiful respite from the week for everyone, but it can also be especially effective for pregnant women. Use it as an excuse to step away from social media for 24 hours and take a break from the constant hit to your self-esteem that comparisons on Instagram can be. Use the day to rest in whatever way heals you. For me, it's vacuuming (I know; I'm weird and technically this isn't a kosher for Shabbat activity); but binge watching Netflix or cuddling in with your dog and a good book works, too.

The biological changes happening within you are physically exhausting and emotionally draining. Many women describe one of the most difficult parts of pregnancy is not feeling like themselves. It is really hard to not have your usual energy, enthusiasm, emotions, energy or appetite. There's a tremendous loss of control that happens in pregnancy: whether you have an easy first trimester, whether you deliver on time, whether you have an easy labor and delivery—it's almost all out of your hands to some degree. You aren't even in charge of when you need to pee, and your hormones can make emotional shifts that much sharper! This is where Judaism steps in and says, wait, you don't need to push yourself to be anything (at least one day a week!).

I realized after the umpteenth doctor's appointment that every aspect of my physical body was 100% devoted to this unborn baby. I had to limit what I ate (No soft cheese! No sushi!) and what I did (No hot tubs! No bike riding!) and I started to really miss some of the things that used to be part of my everyday life. In a way I was really losing myself to the hope and preparation of becoming a mother.

I also felt like doing anything just for me—or rather, this pregnant version of myself—was a waste. After all, it was only going to be a few months; so why bother? So I didn't buy many maternity clothes and I didn't invest in things that were supposed to help (like the pregnancy pillow) because I didn't feel that my pregnant self deserved something for only a few months. I really began to resent my ballooning body and miserable moods and self-care was at an all-time low.

It seemed frivolous to buy all these pregnancy products and I realize looking back that I was living in a mentality of "Wait for the baby to be born; then life can begin!" But, when you think about it, almost everything you're going to buy or do for the baby is only going to be for a few months (the $400 MamaRoo bouncer...) yet none of those adorable baby products seemed frivolous to me. In fact I loved shopping for all of those expensive, useless baby-holding and bouncing things. I treasured them—their packaging, the way they looked in the nursery.

So, I'm advocating that we indulge and invest in our pregnant selves in the same way that we do for our new babies. I started by buying lunch at work more often. Giving myself a break from having to pack lunches was a relief. I also hired a housekeeper to help around the house once a month, and I signed up for a massage package for monthly massages. These are the treats I chose; but find what can help you and *#TreatYoSelf.* It isn't just about money and things (although there are some that can help!); but if it's time or activities that will help, then do what you can to find happiness in these sometimes exhausting and difficult months. After all, as a creator, you have to be nourished and full of life to provide it to others.

Here are some top recommended pregnancy items from all the real moms I interviewed for this book:

- ❏ **Pregnancy pillow**: A pillow specifically designed to help you sleep while pregnant (when most positions are uncomfortable or not allowed) really helps the aches pains and stress on muscles and bones. I found this comfortable for only the second trimester; but some women use it the entire time and find it absolutely essential.
- ❏ **Comfy PJs**: For once in your life, no one expects you to wear jeans that button! Enjoy it and get comfy, because many aspects of pregnancy are uncomfortable—so it's worth finding something you can feel comfortable in. When the baby arrives there will likely be a lot of cameras out snapping photos, so look for PJs you don't mind being photographed in!
- ❏ **Cute maternity clothes**: Without going overboard on this, you should invest in a few key wardrobe staples like black leggings, some cute bump flattering tops, and breathable comfortable dresses if you're pregnant during the summer. There's a connection between feeling good about the way you look and feeling good about yourself in general, and that's really hard

to achieve when **nothing** fits or flatters.

- ❏ **A water bottle**: Water is the **best** thing for pregnant women and is essential to staying healthy and hydrated during a time when your body is building a water-based home for your baby. A nice water bottle you enjoying taking around with you can be really helpful in encouraging you to *drink, drink, drink*.

- ❏ **Massage**: A prenatal massage is a great way to ease pain and stiffness from pregnancy and to encourage healthy blood circulation. Research the business and your massage therapist to ensure they know how to properly perform a massage on a pregnant woman. You should never be lying on your stomach or flat on your back. They should make use of side-lying positions and give you a pillow to keep between your knees to help your body stay aligned.

- ❏ **Mani/Pedi**: If a massage is out of your budget, go for a manicure and/or pedicure (who can reach their toes at this stage anyway!) which comes with a lovely short massage. There is an old wives' tale that certain pressure points stimulated during a pedicure can trigger labor, so do be cautious toward the end of your third trimester.

- ❏ **Housekeeper**: Housework can be a form of healthy aerobic exercise (I find making the bed while pregnant about equivalent to completing a triathlon) but it can also be exhausting and nearly impossible, especially in the later months of pregnancy. Hiring someone to help out even just once a month to tackle the deep cleaning can be really helpful. Some cleaning products contain harsh chemicals that are unsafe for pregnant women, so leave that kind of cleaning to someone else.

- ❏ **Healthy food**: It can be expensive to be healthy, and be costly in terms of time and effort. Fresh fruits and vegetables take time to cut and cook and have a short shelf life. But if you're paying less for a hamburger than a pack of gum, what do you think you're really eating?

- ❏ **Netflix**: I binge watched Gilmore Girls during labor* with my first son and it was a fantastic use of down time. (*I was on an epidural.) Finding a lighthearted series to get lost in can be a great way to zone out of pregnancy stress.
- ❏ **Podcasts**: This one can be free and another great stress reliever to take your mind off baby stress. Going for a walk while listening to a podcast will give you twice the stress relieving benefit; even listening in bed before you fall asleep is a good idea if your mind tends to race.
- ❏ **Pregnancy Photoshoot**: These can be pricey if you go with a professional, but taking time to celebrate your body at this special moment in time can do wonders for your self-esteem. If you find a good photographer they will make you and your bump glow!

One of the mothers I spoke with, Rachel, has three children—three, six, and nine years old. She has some great approaches to parenting, and she shared this advice: The best thing to keep in mind when you're pregnant is not to try to be *SuperMom*! Especially if you have other little ones running around the house, it's OK to take a nap instead of tidying the house. Cut yourself some slack and remember it's going to be OK—you're growing a human! When she was pregnant she treated herself to naps and prenatal yoga!

Another mother I spoke with, Shira, has a six-year-old, a four-year-old and just gave birth to a newborn. Shira said prioritizing a pedicure really helped her. It was a component of preventative care as well as a moment every few weeks where she indulged in a treat for herself. She also benefited from prenatal massage!

The first trimester: real, raw and exposed!
Did you know that if your mother experienced morning sickness, then you will likely experience it too? So in a way your pregnancy experiences are passed down from generation to generation, or *l'dor*

vador in Hebrew—what a very Jewish concept!

The first trimester comprises twelve (at times hellish) weeks of your first exposure to pregnancy. You've seen the second line on the pregnancy test and you've been to see your doctor. Now that the initial excitement is over, the first few weeks of pregnancy begin in earnest. It usually isn't long before your body starts to just feel different (exhausted, sensitive, nauseous). My mom told me she could tell I was pregnant at week four because I just "looked tired"!

I suffered from excruciating morning sickness in my first trimesters and prayed to God every night to help me wake up and feel relief. The nausea was so all-consuming I almost quit my job because I physically couldn't bring myself to get up and go to the office every day. There's also the added pressure of no one knowing you're pregnant and trying to hide how terrible you're feeling. In the end I told my boss what was going on and she encouraged me to keep working but to just take it easy. Many women are not so fortunate.

I personally felt betrayed by my body. I had wanted to be pregnant and have children so badly that I would often fantasize about what the experience would be like. I pictured myself in beautiful maternity clothes, "glowing" just as it had always been described to me. I was blown away and incredibly disappointed in my pregnancy experience. Weeks on end of utter exhaustion all day coupled with unending nausea without any relief. WTF! My doctor told me pregnancy was a wellness and not an illness which was a lovely thought, but that wasn't at all how it felt to me.

I was angry, disappointed, and jealous of all the women on Instagram who had it better than I did. But I took it as a defining moment of understanding the human body—the randomness of sickness and the blessing of health. As the weeks slowly edged onward, I regained some strength and energy and the nausea gradually lifted. I never got "good" at being pregnant; in fact my third time around was the hardest one yet. And I gave up my dream of having a house full of five children because I couldn't physically bear it. I couldn't physically bear them.

But that is the nature of our existence, and I leaned on God more as a source of empathy than comfort. He was my spiritual punching bag I could complain to endlessly about my suffering. And after having it out with Him I'd often come around and thank Him for the ability to get pregnant in the first place and the gift of motherhood. That's my spiritual first trimester, but I encourage anyone suffering to reach out to the spiritual and ask for help, even if you're met with silence. Learning to ask and learning to know your feelings is a gift of its own.

Rabbi Dara Frimmer of Temple Isaiah in West Los Angeles shared her thoughts with me on what the experience of becoming pregnant can really feel like for a woman. She described pregnancy as a "heightened experience of recognizing our body's vulnerability." We tend to go through life, especially when we're young and in our healthiest days, taking for granted all the ways our body has to function. Rabbi Frimmer explained that the experience of being really sick versus living a generally healthy life makes us hyper-aware of our physical body and its functions. The fear that our body isn't working the way it should, and gratitude for the miracle of recovery tends to put things in focus. Similarly, pregnancy can be what I would describe as the ultimate lesson in the vulnerability of our body. No matter how fit and healthy you are, pregnancy can be a debilitating experience for the body or it can be blissful—and ultimately we don't have much choice in that.

Rabbi Dara shared that for her, pregnancy was a miracle, but also a really scary experience. Judaism helped her celebrate and helped provide her comfort, and find the words to offer thanks and gratitude. Through her experience during pregnancy she figured out how to allow her Judaism to be with her through the uncertainty of pregnancy.

One of the women I spoke to, Katie, gave birth to her first child last year, and had some advice for pregnant women. "When I talk to expectant moms now, I tell them that everything everyone told them is a lie! Being pregnant is **not** fun or beautiful! It is nine months of swollen feet, heartburn, never being able to get into a comfortable sleeping position, having to rethink how to put on your clothes and how to use the bathroom and how to shower, and wanting an Italian sub more than you have ever wanted one in your life simply because you cannot have one."

Let's talk tired

For a fun little Friday post on my Instagram I shared that I had been 'woman-splaining' to my husband how exhaustion from pregnancy is unlike just being "tired." I put out a question on my Stories and asked people to tell me how they would describe what pregnancy tiredness felt like, here are a few of my favorite responses:

"5 hours after 5 hour energy"

"Like you've run a marathon and somebody asks you to do laundry, make dinner, and bathe the kids"

"A hurting kind of tired, you can feel through your whole body almost like a pain"

"Like you've got an IV drip of Benadryl"

"Energy depletion"

"Constant hangover"

"A man having a cold"

"Driving your car 40 miles when your tank says 5 left"

"A deflated balloon"

The point is that when women feel tired they sometimes judge themselves a little too harshly. I heard women I interviewed for this book tell me they felt guilty for being so "lazy." This is the furthest thing from the truth. Your body's working overtime, it's literally supporting two lives and it is incredibly physically exhausting even if you haven't done anything else all day, you have spent a day creating a life. Don't take that task lightly or judge your body harshly; it is working as hard as it can.

Take a bath, and take a ritual bath, too

Taking a bath can be a soothing, comforting and healing experience for a pregnant woman's body and mind (so long as the water isn't too hot). In Judaism, women immerse in a ritual bath call the mikvah for similar self-care reasons. The mikvah provides a physical and spiritual experience that is unlike anything else in Jewish observance. It's such an ancient tradition and in a way it combines the tranquility of a modern day spa with the mystical power of a natural body of water. Women who experience it for the first time often describe it as a way to shut the world out for a moment and connect to God and to themselves.

Water is universally cleansing, and there's a centuries-old mystical connection of purity to water. Traditionally women observe the mitzvah of the mikvah many times in a typical year: after each period, before Yom Kippur, and before significant life events like a wedding. *Halachah* (Jewish law) mandates that the mikvah be used in conversion ceremonies, before a woman marries, and in observation of *niddah* (abstaining from sex during her menstrual cycle). But the power of the mikvah experience can be transcending; and as such, Jewish women have found various reasons to partake in this very ancient ritual. Many women today use the mikvah as a way to observe milestones in their lives like graduation or bat mitzvah, or even as a healing tool for separation, divorce, bereavement, or after a miscarriage.

What to expect at a mikvah

If you've never seen a mikvah, the best way I can describe most modern ones is that they look and feel like a spa! There is a room where you get ready to immerse, with instructions on how to immerse in the pool and the traditional prayers to say. There is also a mikvah attendant who can help you and answer your questions. Most mikvahs will have a website where you can see what the facility looks like. Many mikvah attendants will wait outside so you can experience the mikvah privately; but if you're concerned about, this feel free to ask before you go.

A mikvah (pronounced MICK-vuh and can also be spelled *mikveh*), is a Jewish ritual bath. According to Jewish law it must contain enough water within the bath to cover the entire body. To meet the requirements of a kosher mikvah, the pool must contain enough water to cover the entire body of an average sized person (Babylonian Talmud, Eruvin 4b) which the rabbis have calculated to be 40 *seah* (which modern day interpretations note as 150 gallons). The other physical component of mikvah water is that it must be connected to a naturally flowing source or well of naturally occurring water. Today's mikvahs are clean, hygienic and often beautiful places for spiritual immersion.

There are all sorts of mikvahs and therefore many types of mikvah experiences. If this will be your first time going, it's helpful to select one that you will be comfortable with and to let them know that this is your first time so the attendants can help guide you through. The Conservative and Reform movements have many mikvahs that are designed to help people who have never been before and are there for a special occasion, like before getting married or becoming pregnant.

When you arrive you'll be greeted by the mikvah attendant who will explain where everything is and what you need to do. Some mikvahs have a policy that requires an attendant to witness the mitzvah of immersion; others do not. You can ask beforehand if they will accompany you into the mikvah. There is also usually a fee or suggested donation for using the mikvah—usually from between 18 to 36 dollars; but it can be more.

There will be a separate bathroom and washing area with a toilet, sink and shower. This is the preparation area where you'll go through the physical steps before bathing in the mikvah. You should take your time here and use the physical preparation as a mental one as well: slow down, think about why you are there and what you hope to gain from the experience. Perhaps it's just a moment to reflect on the life you're hoping to create, or the health and happiness of yourself or your child that you would like to pray for. You'll go to the bathroom, shower, comb your hair, clean your fingernails and remove every piece of clothing and jewelry.

When you are ready, you'll say a prayer before entering the actual mikvah. The mikvah bath will be a large tub of water, usually warm and very pleasant to submerge in. If the mikvah requires the attendant to be present they will have a way for you to let them know that you are ready to enter and have finished the preparations. This will be an otherwise private experience and though you will be naked, you shouldn't feel uncomfortable (they've seen it all before, probably hundreds of times!). If you are shy, you should let them know and they will know how to make the situation right for you. You will then hand them your towel (or hang it up yourself) before walking down the stairs to enter into the waters. Personally I have always asked the attendant to wait outside as I am fairly shy and get distracted easily.

The rooms are generally low lit; some have candles and have a serene quality. Most will offer prayers written out for you to use, but you can also bring your own. The most essential component of the mitzvah is actually submerging in the water without touching anything. It helps to tuck your body into a ball and force yourself, gently, completely underneath the surface of the water. This is actually a little tricky, the first time I used the mikvah I had to hold my nose and really figure out the mechanics of it all, but that was fine.

There are two customs when it comes to when to submerge and recite the blessings. Sephardic Jews generally recite the blessing first and then submerge, whereas Ashkenazic Jews will submerge once, recite the blessing and then submerge two more times. The first blessing is the same for whatever purpose you are going to the mikvah, the translation here is from the Mayyim Hayyim:

בָּרוּךְ אַתָּה אֲדֹנָי אֱלוֹהֵינוּ מֶלֶךְ הָעוֹלָם,
אֲשֶׁר קִדְּשָׁנוּ בְּמִצְוֹתָיו וְצִוָּנוּ עַל הַטְּבִילָה

Baruch ata adonai eloheinu melech ha-olam asher kid-shanu b'mitz-vo-tav v'tzi-vanu al ha-tevilah.

Blessed are You, Adonai, Ruler of the Universe, Who has sanctified us with mitzvot and commanded us concerning immersion.

It is common to revisit the mikvah again at nine months into your pregnancy, just before the baby is due. Rabbi Danielle Gobuty Eskow President and Founder of OnlineJewishLearning.com talked to me about her beautiful experience with this tradition. The metaphysical component of being submerged in water while also knowing her baby soon to be born was submerged in the water of the womb was transformative for her.

Maharat Ruth of Temple Ohev Shalom in Washington, D.C. explained to me the belief that it's lucky to immerse in the mikvah after someone who has just immersed in their last month of pregnancy. Often synagogues will connect women who are looking to go afterwards or someone in their last month who is offering for someone to follow them. There are no set blessings that must be performed but it is customary for women to say personal prayers to ask for good blessings to become pregnant themselves and to have an easy delivery and a healthy and happy baby.

Personally, the concept of immersing in the mikvah before beginning to conceive or after finding out that I was pregnant and then again at nine months is a very full circle experience. It's a spiritual way to bookend a very physical experience and bring my mind back to a place of self-care and reflection. The mikvah can be a truly private and meditative experience; each time I go there is a sense of immense awe.

Jewish meditation and the spiritually
nutritious benefits of mindfulness

One of the most important ways to care for your body and soul during pregnancy is to care for your mind. The mind-body connection is perhaps most apparent during pregnancy. If you've been lucky enough to live a generally healthy and happy life, pregnancy can be the first time your mind has to relinquish a bit of control to your body. This is the reality of shifting hormones, appetite and energy while growing a human being. Pregnancy can mean feeling extremely tired and drained, both emotionally and physically. Hormones fluctuate, and the sheer physical task of so much cell reproduction can really affect a mother-to-be's mental state.

There is much ongoing research into postpartum depression and prenatal depression, and why some women are more vulnerable than others; a lot is still unknown. What is known is that pregnancy and new motherhood can be a wonderful but stressful time, even for those in the best circumstances. Practicing meditation is actually an ancient Jewish tradition, and the benefits of calming and centering the mind can serve to take back some of that control you may feel like you're losing in your first trimester. I learned the benefits of meditation after my son was born and I wanted to share the uniquely Jewish aspect of meditation that I learned to practice.

I had always wanted to be someone who meditates, just like I wanted to be someone who ran marathons and never ate processed food. Mediation seemed unattainable and wonderful at the same time. Well, let me tell you, unlike other forms of physical well-being, you don't have to move for this one; you can sit on the floor of your own house and successfully meditate. I personally choose my closet, where I can close the door and not be distracted.

One of the things that really kept me from meditating was that everything I read about how to meditate was based on Eastern, usually Buddhist, religious philosophy. A lot of mediation experts will tell you that though Eastern religion inspired a lot of current-day meditation practices, you don't need to practice Buddhism to meditate. The problem for me was that I sort of wished I was Buddhist; as if I believed in the Buddha I would be able to connect to the meditation—the phrases, the chanting, etc. I wanted to feel a spiritual connection to it, but felt unable to because the spiritual connection I had to God was through Judaism.

I started to wonder if I had a way to connect Judaism and meditation I might find some success. I have attended a Shabbat Yoga class, and this was the perfect blend of what I was searching for through meditation. We sang the Friday night kabbalat Shabbat service while doing yoga (very new age, I know!) and it was just so beautiful and spiritual.

I like to say I was trained to pray: I went to Jewish day school and grew up fairly religious, attending services in synagogue almost every Friday night. I love the songs, melodies and community of these familiar experiences. Certain words in certain prayers always stand out to me and really leave me in awe when I consider their meaning. For me that was the key—to meditate on those Jewish phrases and find my spiritual connection to meditation.

I also read a book which helped tremendously, called, of all things, *A Practical Guide to Jewish Meditation*—which was exactly what I was looking for. Rabbi Arye Kaplan, the author, walks you through not only the ancient history of Jewish meditation but also provides a real step-by-step guide to teach anyone how to do it.

I think learning to calm one's mind is a genuine way to take care of your spirit and mind during pregnancy, and to address all the anxiety and stress that can come with it. So if you haven't tried meditation—and especially if you haven't because it never seemed very Jewish—I highly encourage you to give it a go!

One of the methods Rabbi Kaplan discusses is to choose a singular phrase or line of prayer from Jewish text. I chose the last line of the Adon Olam prayer, which I translate as *In his hands I place my soul, when I wake and when I sleep, God is with me I am not afraid.* This is not an exact translation as I wanted to use words that felt like normal speech to me that I could easily repeat. I actually had the very last line of this text *God is with me I am not afraid* inscribed on a necklace that I bought in Israel when I was younger, so the choice was fairly instinctive to me when I was thinking about which line to choose. Then after going through a standard calming exercise of relaxation (there are tons of them out there; I personally like to think about and sense each part of my body from the top of my head to the bottom of my feet until I feel relaxed), I just repeat this one line of prayer. Sometimes I'll visualize myself writing it out in sand, or carving it into a rock, or reading it in a book; whatever it is, I just focus on it.

Other thoughts come and go, sometimes it can be minutes before I'm back to my mini mantra line, but it doesn't matter! It still counts! All you need to do is sit quietly and focus. What you think about and where your mind goes doesn't mean you're not doing it right. So go forth—to your closet, to your favorite comfy chair, to a mountaintop—whatever works for **you,** and try it out!

Let's be real: sometimes pregnancy sucks!
Morning sickness and exhaustion

There are some unfair expectations out there today—especially among the Pinterest and Instagram crowds—that pregnancy is a bunch of magical months of rainbows and unicorns. There are posts from beautiful women, all put together with makeup and adorable outfits announcing their pregnancy, sharing their gender reveals, attending their showers, etc. The onslaught of this imagery can leave a false impression that everyone enjoys pregnancy and lives their best life during these months of great anticipation and expectation.

Jewish superstitions around pregnancy involves a lot of *Don't ask, don't tell* during the first few months (which we'll dive deep into later in this book!). One benefit of this custom is that Jewish moms often don't have to deal with the added pressure of making their pregnancies "glow" for the world around them. Jewish tradition is very focused on protecting a woman who is in the early stages of pregnancy—both spiritually from the *evil eye* and physically from the demands of life.

#DYK? Pregnant Jewish women traditionally do not go to cemeteries or funerals so as not to bring emotional distress or thoughts of death to a developing baby.

If you are feeling nauseous just reading this right now, skip this paragraph—because here is some hard truth from someone who experienced a very common but very unpleasant first trimester of pregnancy. I suffered through weeks on end of nausea and debilitating exhaustion. The struggle was all too real. What was really hard for me to deal with (beyond the symptoms described above) was that women are expected to hide the fact that they're pregnant from the world. I felt like I was hiding something and suffering in silence because it was "too early" to tell my friends, family and coworkers what was really going on. Keeping up with a social life, a home life and, of course, office life is a near impossibility for many women.

The first trimester can be a profound and prolonged exercise in stamina and tolerance. My best advice is to accept your body's reaction to the hormones and changes of pregnancy. Don't fight it, try not to hate it, and don't ignore it. Just listen to your body begging you to rest and to drink water and forget about living up to some fake ideal of what pregnancy should be. Let others take care of you when they offer to help. And if they don't offer—ask!

Top tips for surviving morning sickness

❏ **Rest**: *Yah duh*, if only I had the time! Right. Well, listen—you don't have a choice; your body will always win. If you decide to skip out on what your body is telling you you need, you will just be that much more exhausted and frustrated by life. It is *really* weird to suddenly go from the type of person who works a full-time job, comes home at night to prep their Blue Apron gourmet meal, and then goes out with their partner for a drink and a movie to someone who literally can't make it up the stairs to their bedroom to pass out at 8:00 pm. It's really disorienting, especially since nothing on the outside of your body has changed. It makes sense to be tired and moody when you're eight months pregnant, people get that; but it's actually just as hard for some women during months one and two! There may not even be a hint of a bump yet, but those hormones inside of you are in full pregnancy mode and there's really no fighting them. Yes, it is perfectly normal and natural to feel utterly exhausted in the first few weeks of pregnancy. And as a Jewish woman you should know how important the idea of Shabbat—rest—is to our lives. Many women are more nauseous in the morning (unless you are one of those magical fairies who wakes up feeling refreshed and rejuvenated; if so—HOW??) and at night, when they are the most tired. Exhaustion exacerbates nausea.

- ❏ **Water**: Buy a cute water bottle and a stainless steel straw and get your drink on. Try ice cold water. If you can't stomach water, add flavor drops to it. Other good options are flavored seltzers and tart fruit juices. Try to avoid added sugar when possible. If you are drinking all day your body will be hydrated—which helps ease morning sickness and exhaustion.

- ❏ **Mints & Gum**: This can be very soothing for nausea, and since morning sickness can last for hours and it's hard to eat crackers for hours on end, chewing gum or sucking on mints can really help. Small pieces may be best: large pieces of gum that produce a lot of saliva can make it hard to swallow! Candy canes also work great.

- ❏ **Ginger**: Ginger candies, ginger chews, raw ginger in tea... you get the idea.

- ❏ **Peppermint Tea**: This can soothe your stomach, and it's also helpful if your sinuses are blocked up. For a super sinus clearing drink, make your tea with broth brewed from fresh ginger root.

❏ **Crackers, Pretzels and Toast**: Bland, baby, bland. I even kept these on my bedside table because having a mini snack when I was waking up at night to pee helped the nausea in the morning—an empty stomach can really trigger severe nausea.

❏ **Fruit**: Nice cold fruit can be really helpful. It's packed with nutrients, but it's also packed with **water,** so it can help with hydration. Caution: fruit can have a lot of sugar in it, so moderate yourself accordingly.

❏ **Small frequent meals**: Being hungry and being full both exacerbate morning sickness, so go for small light frequent meals.

❏ **Walk**: I don't want to say that you can just distract yourself from morning sickness, but a breath of fresh air and some physical exercise can at least alleviate a bad spell for a little while. Sometimes I felt unable to get out of bed; but if I actually walked around outside I ended up being able to do the whole neighborhood loop and I felt better during those 20 minutes than if I had spent them wallowing in misery—which I did enough of!

5.
Genetic Testing and Finding out the Gender

Time to get scientific...and emotional. As is so apropos of pregnancy, maternal fetal care is a bizarre mashup of the biology of genetics and the female body intertwined with spirituality, ethics, and emotion. Every prenatal checkup is a perfect showcase of this. Your doctor usually begins each appointment with the obvious question, "So, how are you feeling?"

How you may be feeling about your body and your baby all play into the decisions you need to make during pregnancy. There are women who prefer minimal intervention and choose to leave whoever is growing in their womb undisturbed until they choose to arrive. On the other end of the spectrum are women who want every test and ultrasound available to have as much medical information about their body and their baby as possible. Jewish women fall within every line of this colorful scientific ethical rainbow.

Judaism puts one thing above all else: the preservation of life (or in Hebrew, *pikuach nefesh*). Every Jewish law is subordinate to this divine ideal. However, you might be surprised to know that in many situations Judaism puts the life and preservation of the mother's life above that of the fetus. Before we get into the most complicated and ethical concepts of pregnancy, let's start simple.

Building on the concept of *pikuach nefesh*, Judaism encourages women to have complete prenatal care and maternal fetal medical care. The recommendation of a doctor is almost always paramount over that of a rabbi. Jewish culture places a high value on the art and ability to care and heal, which could be why there are a lot of Jewish doctors!

There is generally little *halachic* (Jewish legal) objection to the use of ultrasound examinations during pregnancy. The procedure is safe and non-invasive, and above all, almost any rabbi will tell you that if your doctor recommends something, you should follow their advice. So if your OB schedules ultrasounds at certain weeks of the pregnancy, then that is when you should have them. Regular medical care and ultrasounds are essential to keep both mom and baby healthy.

In the 1980s the Chabad Rebbe spoke out against routine early ultrasounds due to the number of false alarms doctors were observing that may have contributed to abortions when the fetus would have otherwise developed normally. Today ultrasounds are routine even among the religious Orthodox women. Still the historical legacy that *Jewish women don't get ultrasounds* has persisted in some communities despite its inaccuracy.

Should you undergo genetic testing?

When it comes to medical intervention in pregnancy, like most things in Judaism—and here is probably the most trite concept in the whole book—only *you* can decide what is best for you.

There are some research statistics that show more Jewish women are getting intervention testing done in pregnancy. In a paper titled "Increasing rates of prenatal testing among Jewish and Arab women in Israel over one decade," the authors found that of a total of 569 Jewish women in Israel interviewed, there was an increase in the rate of early screenings—including nuchal translucency tests and amniocentesis—in the past decade. The authors found that prenatal testing was becoming more popular among Jewish women, especially those who had higher income and medical insurance.

Many leaders in the Jewish community advocate for genetic carrier screening before a couple decides to get pregnant—or even decides to get married—so they are aware of the potential risks of pregnancy. Many diseases are more prevalent within the Jewish community, due in part to a small insular population and to the "bottlenecking" that occurred after the Holocaust, reducing genetic diversity. Fatal diseases like Tay Sachs are common within the Jewish Ashkenazi population, and other diseases have a higher incidence in the Jewish community than in the national population.

Many authorities in the Jewish and medical community today advocate for genetic screening and gene therapy, because in the Torah we are commanded to heal the sick. There are many writings from great Jewish philosophers like Rashi who analyze stories in the Torah where someone was hurt or injured; contemporary Jewish thinkers take from that a core Jewish principle that advancements in science and healing are a mitzvah. The use of genetic testing and intervention is a way of healing these debilitating diseases within the community.

In the 1970s, due to the devastating number of Jewish children born with the fatal Tay-Sachs disease, the Jewish community successfully mobilized prescreening for couples and virtually eradicated the disease. Thanks to the commitment of community organizers and advancements in scientific technology, Jewish couples have more health screening options today than just a few decades ago.

Couples today are permitted by Jewish rabbis to use in vitro fertilization (IVF) and prescreening of zygote embryos to take precautions to ensure the best chance of a healthy life for their future children. There are even cases where rabbinic authorities have approved choosing the sex of one's baby if there is a concern about gender-specific genetic diseases.

Genetic testing for diseases prevalent in the Jewish community

Today, companies like JScreen are vocal in advocating prescreen testing. I spoke to Hilary Kenner, the Director of National Outreach for Emory University's JScreen Program, who shared some valuable insight into what genetic screening is and why it's so important for Jewish families (including interfaith and unaffiliated ones!).

JScreen was started in Atlanta (there's a bit of a *trigger warning* on this one). A few years ago, husband and wife Randy and Carol Gold were just a 'normal' Jewish family. Before having children they had been screened by their own doctors for genetic diseases, including the 'Ashkenazi Jewish panel' (which screens for diseases common in this community). Each of their genetic screening tests came back normal and they went on to get pregnant. Their first child was born healthy; but their second child showed early signs of something being wrong. The baby girl had low muscle tone and was behind on her milestones. After much heartbreak, doctors' visits and medical tests it was revealed that she had been born with a rare and devastating genetic diagnosis: ML4. The couple were shocked. How could this have happened when they both had been tested?

The truth is that most genetic screening covered by insurance and offered through your doctor's office is, unfortunately, very limited. Even having the traditional "Ashkenazi panel" offered in many doctors' offices doesn't cover everything. The Gold family took their struggle and grief and launched JScreen. Through the support of generous donations, the organization now offers couples comprehensive genetic testing that is easy and affordable.

According to JScreen, only 24% of young Jews have heard of these tests or have been screened. No one was telling them to go out and do this—not their doctors, not their rabbis, not their parents. JScreen only launched in 2013, but already it has gained tremendous momentum in the Jewish community.

So...how much is it? Normally, genetic testing is very expensive, running about $1,000 when not covered by insurance. JScreen kits are just $149 and are mailed right to your home. They screen for over 200 diseases (about half of which are more common in Ashkenazi, Sephardi or Mizrah Jewish populations—even with just one Jewish grandparent), which is incredibly comprehensive. It's important for both partners to be screened, even if one of the partners isn't Jewish! Just because a disease is prevalent within the Jewish population doesn't mean that a person who isn't Jewish can't be a carrier.

Also, remember: carriers are normal healthy individuals!

One the most important components of JScreen is that when you complete your kit, you are matched to a genetic counselor. The genetic counselor is a real person (not just a screen chat-bot) available to talk about your results, present best options and next steps, and to connect you with resources in your area. There are many options for couples who are carriers. Screening positive for a disease isn't an end to their conception journey; it's a real beginning of a chance to have a healthy baby. Each pregnancy is an independent risk; so even if you have had a healthy child, it's important to be tested before adding to your family. Science continues to advance and screening is likely to become more sensitive.

I asked Hilary, what if you're scared? She told me; knowledge is power. "You wouldn't cross the street without looking both ways would you?" she asks. Genetic screening works on the same principle. Screening offers us a chance to do what we can for our future kids. One mom I spoke with is Erin; she recently gave birth to a beautiful baby girl. Erin said her rabbi told her and her husband about the JScreen program and that her synagogue even helped cover the cost of the test. If you have concerns about the cost or how the test works, go to JScreen.org for more information! The tests are mailed directly to you with comprehensive information on how the test works and how to collect the saliva sample for screening.

Terminating a pregnancy

(Some of this information is also in Chapter 2. Please refer to those pages for more information on healing from terminating a pregnancy.)

Abortion. I doubt there's a word in the English language that stirs up more emotion or controversy than that one. Unlike many of our religious Christian neighbors, most Jews (84%, according to the Pew Religious Landscape Survey) support legalized abortion in all or most cases.

Jewish law does not consider a fetus to be a life of its own until it is born. Although an unborn baby is still precious as it has the potential for life, it is considered a part of the mother's body until it emerges from the womb.

It is for this reason that abortion has been allowed as a means to save the mother's life: if, for example, the pregnancy is putting her life in danger. Today many Jewish thinkers have expanded this message of compassion to the fetus and with genetic testing and advanced early ultrasounds also allow for abortions when the child would be born into a life of suffering and pain.

Many rabbis would caution against reading too broadly into this meaning that all abortions are considered ethical, and would advise against relying on abortion as a form of contraception. However, modern Judaism, especially as the Reform, Conservative and Reconstructionist movements live it, is very progressive and empowering of women and their choices regarding their bodies.

OK, let's have some fun now.
Do you want to know the sex of the baby?
Today in modern Jewish communities it is very popular to find out the sex of the baby early on in the pregnancy. However, there are also many families who choose not to know ahead of time or to keep that information a secret. According to Jewish custom, some people will choose not to learn this information based on the midrash that one of the seven things concealed from humanity is what's inside a mother's womb. This secret space is also referred in the Torah: "Just as you do not know how the lifebreath passes into the limbs within the womb of the pregnant woman, so you cannot foresee the actions of God, who causes all things to happen" (Ecclesiastes 11:5).

For my first pregnancy I was so excited to tell my friends and family that we were going to have a boy. My husband and I planned a small celebration for just my immediate family. We were going to bake a *gender reveal* cake and fill the inside with blue sprinkles and candy. My family lives in Los Angeles and we were booked to fly out the next week where the plan was to invite the family over to open the cake with us. Of course, one week before our big gender reveal I was chatting with my mom on the phone while doing my grocery shopping when I mentioned something about the bris...so that was that! Ugh, #facepalm. In my other pregnancies I have done one sort of reveal or another for the sex of the baby and for me they have always been the happiest part of the first trimester. For me there wasn't much else to plan or enjoy during those really rough weeks of exhaustion and nausea, so sharing the *boy* or *girl* news (well for me, it's always *boy*!) was just something that really helped and cheered me up.

I also personally love *gender reveal* surprises; with my being a YouTuber, that shouldn't surprise you. Also, if you're looking for some lighthearted entertainment, search "gender reveal fails" on YouTube; you are in for a laugh!

Many Jewish parents will avoid any grand reveals, though, because of how Judaism views what's the in womb (i.e. not a life of its own yet), and for superstitious reasons. It's also less common among Jewish families to have baby showers or decorate their nurseries until the baby is born. More on that in the next chapter! These however are all customs, and you won't be surprised to find out that the Torah says nothing about gender reveal parties. You might have grandparents or friends against the idea. But if finding out the baby's sex and sharing that information with friends is something that you want to do there is no law in Judaism that says you can't.

6.

B'sha-ah Tova: Sharing the News, and a Note on Superstition

Growing up as the only kid in town without a Christmas Tree is hard enough, but being the only mom on Instagram who doesn't have a baby shower…that's tough, too! Although there is no Jewish law that prohibits celebrating pregnancy or purchasing items for the baby before he or she arrives, there's a lot of superstition surrounding these practices. Judaism is overstuffed with *Bubbe-meise*—a Yiddish term for a hardened cultural superstition. And nowhere is this more apparent than a woman preparing for the birth of a baby.

I've been told that it's kind of strange for someone who wasn't raised in a Jewish home to come to grips with the level of superstition surrounding Judaism and pregnancy. While everyone else is throwing baby showers and decorating nurseries, Jews are speaking in whispers and leaving out words when even mentioning their pregnancy. Why? Well there are some positive aspects to this. First, if a woman did lose a pregnancy she wouldn't have to face a house full of baby gear and a nursery prepared for a baby that would never live to enjoy it. Second, because a developing fetus isn't a full life of its own according to Jewish law, women are empowered with the right to make decisions over their body; this is why so many Jews support female reproductive rights. In an American culture consumed with celebrating all things bump-related, I was curious how these Jewish superstitions began and whether it was worth it to hold onto them.

There is a strong cultural precedence that can be interpreted as a sort of spiritual safety net for pregnant women—who before the advent of modern medicine were likely to see many infant and pre-natal deaths. This same line of thought explains why there aren't Jewish mourning rituals for miscarriage (more on that in Chapter 2).

Even before I became pregnant I knew the rules: Don't say the baby's name. Don't buy anything for the baby. Don't plan a bris (God forbid!). Oh, and don't talk about what life will be like when the baby arrives. Because, of course, the *evil eye* is always watching, and you don't want to tempt fate.

I found out that I would be losing my first pregnancy when I was 5 months along. It didn't make sense. We didn't own a single baby item. We didn't have a registry. I hardly even spoke about the fact that I was pregnant. I had a difficult time spiritually grieving the loss, and I desperately wanted to hold onto something from the pregnancy. To have a physical memento of a child I would never meet. I thought about how if I had just had a blanket embroidered with his name on it, that it would be a nice thing to keep in my nightstand and hold while I wept those many months after the loss.

When, a year later, I gave birth to a healthy baby boy, I arrived home to a state of total disarray. The only baby item we had purchased was the legally required car seat to take the baby home in, and two plain onesies for him to wear. I did have a secret list of items on Amazon that could ship next day once the baby was born. (I hadn't even put them in my online cart, because *kenahora*!) I thought this was a smart practical idea, until we were in the hospital after a slightly traumatic delivery; and instead of being able to be totally present with me, my husband, understandably, was frantically searching online for things like diapers and thermometers on his phone.

The lovely homecoming we've all seen so many photos of on Instagram was instead a jumble of boxes and family members quickly trying to assemble something for the baby to sleep in while I sat on the edge of the bed in my pajamas too exhausted to help or even direct much of the action.

Before I had a baby I would look at nursery tour videos online with the baby's name in big wooden block letters mounted on the wall months before it's even been born and think, "So silly — what are they thinking?" Now I look at those same images and think, "This makes sense. I was an idiot." Nesting is a natural instinct, and

I believe the physical preparation of the home does wonders for putting a nervous mom-to-be's mind at ease.

If I am lucky enough to have more children I will prepare for them however I wish. I'll buy some baby clothes; I'll wash crib sheets and I'll think about the future with hope and happiness in my heart. I've already suffered loss without doing anything to deserve it, and I don't believe bad things happen to good people because they go to *buybuyBaby*.

Rabbi Danielle Eskow of OnlineJewishLearning.com shared a similar experience. Because she had experienced a pregnancy loss, she truly understood how random the event was—there is nothing anyone can do to prevent it. So when she became pregnant again, she celebrated every moment of that pregnancy. Her refusal to bend to superstitions was a way of rising above them. She even had a baby shower and decorated her little girl's nursery.

One nice counterpoint to this perspective was offered to me by Rabbi Stutman, who knows that really—when you bring the baby home, you don't *need* all 150 items recommended on the "must-have" baby list at every baby supplies superstore. European countries are bucking the consumerist trend and sending women home from the hospital with a cardboard box (an extremely safe place for a newborn to sleep) and a handful essential items to clothe and diaper the baby.

Jewish superstition can help pregnant parents avoid the temptation to blow the baby budget on things they'll never need. I personally owned **three** baby swings and **three** infant carriers, but I think that can be attributed to the fact that because I didn't buy anything before my son was born, I might have gone a little overboard when he was finally here.

Rabbi Stutman reminded me that when Jewish communities thrive, they come together to support new parents. They prepare the nursery while new parents recover in the hospital and they set up meal trains and other services to welcome and care for newborns that go beyond "stuff" that has to be purchased in advance.

Baby stores in Jewish areas are aware of these superstitious traditions and serve their clientele by offering full delivery services after the baby is born. Lazar's Furniture in the north end of Chicago, for example, will hold everything at their store until you call with news that the baby is born; then they will assemble and deliver everything to your home.

If you'd like to follow some of the traditional Jewish superstitions about pregnancy here's a short and simple checklist for you:

- ❏ Don't announce your pregnancy in a big public way; wait to share the news with family and friends until you're 4 or 5 months pregnant and it becomes obvious.
- ❏ When someone shares news that they are pregnant the appropriate response is *b'shaah tovah* ("at a good hour"), not Mazal Tov or Congratulations.
- ❏ Don't have a gender reveal celebration.
- ❏ Don't have a baby shower.
- ❏ Don't decorate the nursery or bring any baby items into the house before the baby is born.
- ❏ Wear a red ruby charm for good luck during pregnancy and labor.
- ❏ Don't visit a cemetery or attend a funeral.
- ❏ Don't share publicly any "bump updates" or other pregnancy milestones.
- ❏ Don't reveal the baby's name until the baby has arrived.

Jewish pregnancy superstitions—helpful or harmful?

Rabbi Jaclyn Cohen of Temple Isaiah in West Los Angeles told me that, like many aspects of rituals and observations, the rules (*halachah*) and traditions (*minchag*) of pregnancy are "community-specific and rabbi-dependent"—so much of what a community does is set in motion by its rabbinic leadership. Some synagogues openly celebrate pregnancy, while in other synagogues it is a more private experience—largely due to superstitions surrounding it.

Rabbi Cohen explained that part of this quietness surrounding pregnancy is due to the very real and relevant notion that pregnancies can be lost. Beyond that though, Judaism is also very focused on the next generation and many elements of prayer and our holidays revolve around the idea of *l'dor vador* (from generation to generation). So we focus our customs and rituals on teaching our children so that they can grow and multiply and continue the tradition. She asked me if we are so focused on the next generation that we've lost site of the woman as a person and who she is before she gets to that "finish line" of giving birth.

In some ways all the secrecy and silence and superstition has resulted in a period of isolation and lonely suffering for Jewish women. If we can't share our experiences, how can we learn and be comforted by our community? When a child becomes a bar mitzvah, his growth leading up to his moment of triumph is celebrated. When a couple becomes engaged they too are celebrated from the moment they announce their decision through their arrival at the chuppah. During moments of transition, Judaism is there as we honor life-cycle moments. But where in Jewish learning do we establish that pregnant women and new moms need support and encouragement from the community?

One of the mothers who shared her experience for this book, Erin, said that she followed Jewish superstitious customs "to a point." She told friends and family from the beginning that she did not want a baby shower or baby items in her home. When she got to eight months along she did start purchasing some essentials, like the car seat and a few items for the baby's room. She said the custom of not sharing the baby's name early meant that she didn't feel stressed about the fact that she and her husband hadn't decided on one yet!

Beth, like many of the Jewish mothers I interviewed for this book, told me that superstition played a major role in her pregnancy. She said, "My mom and grandmothers (who were both living) were very superstitious. I did pick out a layette but did not bring anything into the house. My mom was a big believer in red ribbons to keep away the evil spirits. She put them on my hospital bag, delivery bed and under the mattress." Beth said she embraced this and it helped her feel her family's love and caring.

Maharat Ruth of Ohev Shalom Synagogue Washington, D.C. told me that although the Jewish families in her congregation still remain superstitious, some things, like learning the gender of their baby before they're born, is common. And while the superstitions are still top of mind, some people find them just so impractical that they do end up buying some baby items even if they do feel a little bit guilty about it.

This is a #HOTtopic among Jewish women today and I'm not surprised if you have different thoughts or reactions to the debate. The good news is, Judaism grows, expands, and changes each generation—but the core values stay intact. Whichever side of the superstition debate you fall on, the important thing is to keep the discussion going!

When to share your happy news

In the first few months of pregnancy there can be a push and pull of emotions, wanting to hide and wanting to show. I know I searched "pregnancy bump photos" on Pinterest because I really wanted to know when I would start to show. Turned out for my subsequent pregnancies no searching was required—pretty much right away!

I also had many conversations with my husband about when we should reveal the news. These days if a girl skips a drink at a party or orders her eggs well done at brunch she might as well just post an ultrasound photo; but there's also a hesitancy to share good news until you're *sure* the news is good. But when can you ever really be sure?

After finding out I was pregnant, I felt a strong internal conflict: I wanted to hide and disguise what I felt was very private news, and at the same time I wanted to tell everyone what was happening.

Sometimes your body may make the news more public than you'd initially like it to be. I had really bad morning sickness and ended up telling friends and family early on because I really needed their support and understanding for why I was suddenly a human blob who couldn't get off the couch. I'd rather have them understand and be sympathetic instead of thinking I was a flake. I also strategically only told people I wouldn't mind telling if something did go wrong—or rather, people I'd want to know so they could support me if it did.

I knew there were others who knew without me saying anything, colleagues at work who weren't totally oblivious to my needing to escape every so often (to lie down in my car), my constant snacking, and my ever-expanding waistline. But even if you think people might already know, it's **your** choice to announce it and it's rare that folks will pointedly ask before you tell them, which is nice.

It's entirely up to **you** when you'd like to share your happy news that you're expecting. If you're interested in the Jewish customs around this you'll find a wide variety of opinions. In religious communities, Jewish women don't announce a pregnancy in the traditional American way and are hesitant to even tell anyone they are pregnant before the fifth month. Some Jewish scholars believe this 40-day mark is when the baby receives its soul.

In more modern and liberal communities, you will see lots of announcements on Facebook and myriad adorable "we're expecting" photos. Most Jewish women do wait until after the first 12 weeks of pregnancy and the end of the first trimester before sharing their news publicly because this is when the likelihood of miscarriage decreases.

My advice is to share your happy news with those whom you would also share your sad news. If the worst does happen and your pregnancy ends in a miscarriage or early loss, you may be thankful to have told people so they can be there to support you in dark times. However, if that seems like it would be too much unnecessary pressure, then you definitely don't need to.

When we lost a pregnancy, we were quite far along and had already announced our news; at that point I was sporting a rather large bump, so there wasn't really any hiding it. For the few weeks afterwards I still looked pregnant and not everyone knew what had happened. This resulted in some especially awkward elevator conversations at work. That being said, I definitely didn't regret sharing the news because we had an outpouring of support when it happened and it truly lifted our family up with love and support.

If the worst does happen, I don't believe you should ever feel embarrassed or guilty in any way. You didn't tempt fate and you didn't do anything to be ashamed of. If you were powerful enough to determine if a potential life grows to live or die you'd probably be using your powers more!

Some Jewish customs say that if you can just be modest enough covering that bump and resist the temptation to share happy news, you won't be smote down by the *evil eye*. Personally, I find this line of thought to be detrimental and to serve as a false sense of control. No one has control over these matters; whatever fate has determined for you and your baby will come to pass, even if you follow every superstition and all of your doctor's guidelines. In fact, most pregnancy losses occur because the fetus did not have the right genetic makeup for a healthy life, not because in week five of the pregnancy the mom whispered her excitement to her friend.

As American Jews, we are strongly influenced by American culture. That's why it's become largely acceptable to go trick-or-treating on Halloween; earlier generations of even fairly secular Jewish children did not mark this holiday because of its Pagan roots, or Valentine's Day because of its Christian roots. American culture has become one of the utter glorification of pregnancy: there are apps with photo stickers to update friends and family with each milestone at each week. They're called #Bumpdates (i.e., Baby Bump Updates) and you could spend the next nine months scrolling through them on Instagram if you like.

So for many Jewish people in America, the superstitions and secrecy around pregnancy and pregnancy announcements have become a conflict of cultures. The joy of celebrating a pregnancy is so tempting; and because there isn't a religious reason not to (unlike Christmas!) there's a generational movement toward a more relaxed and supportive community for pregnant Jewish women. However, there are definitely some Jewish people who will still say it's *goyisha* (a slightly harsh Yiddish term for something non-Jews do) to outwardly share pregnancy news.

Another thing to think about is how to receive pregnancy news from others. When Jewish people do share the happy news that they're expecting, "Mazal Tov" and "Congratulations" are not quite the appropriate responses. One thought on this is that these phrases could tempt the *evil eye*. Another reason behind this practice is that saying Mazal Tov implies that the cause for celebration is already here; in Judaism the belief is that isn't the case until the baby arrives. Instead the traditional response is "b'sha-ah tova!"—which translates from Hebrew to "in a good hour," but means something more to the effect of "I hope everything happens when the timing is right." Phrases like *b'sha-ah tova* are all part of this Jewish pregnancy language and culture created in the hopes of protecting parents from disappointment if the pregnancy ends early.

Observing other Jewish pregnancy customs

Many Jewish customs and superstitions about pregnancy are just that, and not law. There are no Jewish laws or ancient rabbinic rulings that certain practices are to be avoided. Here's a female empowerment thought on this: women possess a miraculous—maybe divine— knowledge about themselves and their bodies. If you're conflicted, follow your intuition.

Visiting a cemetery

Jewish pregnant women generally avoid going to a cemetery, even when a relative has passed away. As this is not a Jewish law and just a tradition, it is totally up to you whether or not you want to go to a funeral or visit the cemetery. A good general rule of thumb is that if it is more distressing **not** to go, then you should go. For example, if an immediate family member or a very close friend passed away you might consider going, because not going would cause you even more anguish. You may get some stares or unwanted comments from the older generation though, so be warned! Another option is to attend the funeral but not the burial, or just the shivas but not any of the events where the body would be present.

This custom stems from the notion that when one is creating life, it is best to avoid being near death. Custom says that a baby in his mother's womb is affected by the outside world, both physical and spiritual. Part of this is the connection to a mom's emotions. Mothers, of course, want to create a safe and happy home for the baby during their nine months in the womb, and attending a funeral could cause undue emotional distress for the mother—and therefore the baby as well. This custom also stems from the desire to keep the mom's focus and energy on positive experiences, and away from the sadness of death.

Red Ribbons & Rubies

You've probably seen the red pieces of string that Kabbalah follow-ers (like Madonna, among other mortals) wear tied to their wrists. They also sell these strings at the Western Wall in Jerusalem, and there are some wrapped around Rachel's tomb in Bethlehem. There is also a custom of tying a red ribbon, called in Yiddish a *roite bindele*, to a newborn baby's crib to keep away the *evil eye* or the evil desires of Lilith (Adam's first wife before Eve) and red rubies are said to be lucky fertility charms for women. What's with all this red?

Many scholars believe that Judaism isn't the only culture to have adopted this ancient practice and superstitious connection to the color red. Some rabbis believe that the practice originated outside of Jewish roots and that participating in these practices is prohibited.

Personally I did not grow up knowing of this custom, but my husband's grandmother asked us to place a ribbon under our baby's crib. As you've probably guessed by now, I really don't like superstitions. I rationalized that to me it was just a ribbon and no one could see it; so if it made her happy to know it was there, who was I to object? If you are the type of person who feels connected to the power that may be transferred into these objects then you should feel free to embrace these ancient practices. If all this red feels burdensome to you then follow your own heart on what is meaningful and what is not.

Expecting Jewish!

The Second Trimester

7.

Preparing for Motherhood

*"Mothers need just as much attention as a newborn,
because they too have just been born"*

—Anonymous

Someone is going to call you "Mom"

You've spent months preparing your body for labor and delivery and your home for the arrival of a new baby, but can you ever really be ready to become a mom? Every person experiences this pivotal life shift differently. Personally I was like, "Heck yes, bring it on!" I was already a mom to two dog-babies, after all (only dog moms will appreciate this!) and felt totally comfortable with attending to their daily needs and sacrificing my own time and energy for them. Anyone who has potty trained a puppy on the 11th floor of a city high-rise in a snowstorm gets it. But glimpses of motherhood didn't just occur to me while caring for my dogs; I also felt I had a nurturing tender heart toward my friends and my family. The aspects of motherhood I most admired were the same ones I couldn't wait to further identify with. But that is definitely not always how things work out.

I spoke to many moms who fell somewhere along a spectrum of completely terrified to pretty nonchalant about what parenthood would bring. There were moms who didn't read pregnancy or parenting books because they didn't want to worry about the future, and there were women who hired themselves a full support team (doulas, nannies and various caregivers) to walk them through what they envisioned would be a difficult learning curve. However you are feeling right now, you are not the first—and you are not alone.

I find the power of a mother's intuition to be the most interesting and empowering aspect of how your identity can change when you give birth. It's the one thing you'll have that no one else can claim. You can say, "My baby is tired" and "My baby is hungry," even though everyone in the room might respond, "Oh, but he doesn't look it," or "Oh, but he just ate," and you will always be right. Take pride and strength in that: you will always know your baby best. Not his grandmother; not his nanny; it will always be you. And with that comes the responsibility to defend his needs, and to fight for him when he has no words. Parenthood is an awesome responsibility and I believe that the day you become a mom is the day your instincts and intuitions (if you can learn to listen to them) are born, too.

What makes a good Jewish mother?

Preparing for motherhood is one thing, but how do you prepare to be a good Jewish mom? Motherhood from a Jewish perspective isn't just about mastering a chicken noodle soup recipe (although that's not a bad idea). It's about being prepared spiritually for what taking on this new role in life will mean.

If you're looking for an example of a good Jewish mother, the Torah will point you directly to the matriarch Rachel. In fact, the anniversary of her passing, marked on the 11th of the Hebrew month of Cheshvan, is considered a type of Jewish Mother's Day. Rachel's story of motherhood begins with her suffering for many years with infertility, made that much more painful by her sister Leah's ability to bear children for her husband Jacob. When Rachel did become a mother she was often likened to a mother of all the Jewish people; it is said that she carried a divine presence within her. Her story of mourning for the Jewish people in exile and being told by God that He will return them to their land is one of the foremost examples of her connection to God.

In Jewish tradition it is the mother who protects and sustains religion. She passes her faith along physically (Judaism is a matrilineal religion) and spiritually, as it's her job to nurture a love of Judaism within her home and children.

Raizy Fried (@*Raizyscookin* on Instagram) is a Jewish mother extraordinaire who posts amazing kosher recipes and even better life advice on her Instagram account and website. One post in particular really spoke to me. She had just shared what some will say is the best chocolate cookie recipe out there, and one of her followers commented that they wished they were a "good mom" who had time to bake with her kids.

Raizy took to *Instastories* to share her thoughts on this. She said that a good mom is not someone who bakes with their kids. She explained to her audience that you are not a better mom if you do things like home baking, or a worse one if you don't. If you want to be a good mom, if you have this desire in your heart then guess what? You **are** a good mom. Being a good mom isn't about doing the aesthetic mothering acts that look good on an Instagram square. It's about giving of yourself with kindness and love to your children.

This conversation really hit me. What Raizy was sharing was that if you feel that "mom guilt"—if you even take the time to think about how much you love and care for your children and how much you want to do for them—then you are a good mom.

Expanding on that, though, I believe a good Jewish mom is one who cares and tries to bring the blessings of Judaism into their children's lives. Being a good Jewish mom to me means sharing the Jewish values and traditions that are meaningful to you and creating that same meaning for your children.

Erin, who just had her first child, told me she felt "like I have been preparing my whole life" for motherhood. For her, becoming a Jewish mom is about "modeling behavior such as lighting Shabbat candles or what values you choose to lead your life by." Another mom I spoke to, Daniella, shared that to her it was about giving her children a foundation of faith to give them comfort and community in a big and oftentimes scary world.

There is a lot of bad publicity about the current state of *mommy wars*, the idiotic competition to see whose child reaches which milestones first, and who can avoid screen time the longest. The truth, of course, is that what you're seeing on social media is everyone's best self, edited and retouched to appear as though they always live with soft natural light shining over them. We all know this, but it's still really hard not to be influenced by it. So, my advice: decide what makes a good mom—to you! Write it down—right here, right now—if you want and live by your own code of motherhood.

Your List:

1.

2.

3.

4.

5.

Do you want to hear my list for what makes a good Jewish mother, now that you've written yours? OK, here it is:

1. **Always be kind**. No matter how many times you've asked your child to please, please get in their car seat; no matter how many times you've counted to five before you have to leave the park; no matter how many times you've pleaded to the night sky to just let this baby fall asleep—they are so very little and the world is so very big and they are trying their best just to figure it out, just like you are. So be kind.

2. **Live in the moment**. Judaism has a heightened focus on the present. Life isn't about getting somewhere in the world to come; it's about living **in** the here and now **for** the here and now. Children are the absolute best at this and adults with phones glued to their palms are the absolute worst. The truth is you won't be building Lego towers or having tea parties for long. These little games are infinitely important to your child and if you don't participate in them when you have the chance, that chance will be gone forever (Dramatic much? I know!).

3. **Share a love of learning**. There's a reason Jewish people are called the "People of the Book." Knowledge and the pursuit of it is a traditional Jewish value. Wherever we go, from the grocery store to a stroller walk, we are always learning. I talk to my son about what we see and share everything I know with him. I know he'll get the basics in kindergarten, but I love telling him something new and hearing him share it back to me. On his first day of school I baked him challah in the shape of A, B and C and the Hebrew letters *Aleph*, *Bet* and *Gimmel* and drizzled honey on top, in hopes that learning will always be sweet for him. When I grew up we were given

honey sticks when we embarked on a new chapter of Torah to study.

4. **Share a love of Judaism.** From Shabbat to holiday celebrations, I invest my time and energy in sharing Jewish activities with my son because I believe it's a gift. Wherever his faith goes, as he grows at least I've given him the option to believe in something bigger. We listen to Jewish music in the car and attend Shabbat playgroups, and I try to expose him to all there is to love about our religion.

5. **Make Judaism FUN!** Growing up, it seemed to me that Christians had way more fun than I did; Christmas and Easter especially just seemed so **fun**! With my family, I do indulge in Americanizing some Jewish holidays. For example, on Hanukkah we go all out with eight nights of presents and we decorate the house. For me the goal is to create a celebration that includes the children and creates a holiday they will love. On Passover I create my own Haggadah (using *Haggadot.com*—a great resource!) so that the Seder will be enjoyable for everyone. As my kids grow up I hope the night will conclude with silly plays or skits or whatever they come up with!

Judaism and the art of preparation

Judaism has a lot of traditions surrounding the art of preparation. Before Passover begins we are told to go around our house and seek out all the *chametz* (leavened food forbidden during Passover) and make sure our home is cleaned and ready for the holiday. Before Yom Kippur we must seek forgiveness from those we have wronged. Before Sukkot we must build a sukkah. Before even entering a room we must kiss a mezuzah! There's a lot of *getting ready* when it comes to being Jewish, and many of these physical exercises are a means of creating a spiritual mindset to achieve what we need to when the big moment arrives.

Pregnancy can be a similar practice in preparation, but stretched out over a **much** longer time period. As a result, a lot of pregnancy can feel like a waiting game—a long, long waiting game. If you're in the midst of this feeling, just be thankful you're not an elephant: they have a gestational cycle of nearly two years, and their babies are born weighing an average of 200 pounds!

Rabbi Stutman told me there are so many ways for Judaism to play a role in your life as you prepare for parenthood. When a baby enters the family system it can be a very destabilizing event. Ultimately we don't know who we will bring home from the hospital. Will he be handsome? Will she be athletic? Will the baby even be healthy? Some parents don't even know if they'll be bringing a boy or a girl into their lives.

At this time of the unknown, Jewish ritual can be a comforting source of consistency for a caregiver. For instance, Rabbi Stutman spoke of how the celebration of Shabbat can be a time to take back some control, connect as a family, and find a respite from the outside world and its pressures. Parents ask Rabbi Stutman, "What should we do?" during these long nine months, when *halachically* there really is nothing to do but wait for that baby to arrive. During this waiting time she recommends "building the Jewish life you want to live when your child is here." That can mean figuring out a way to make Shabbat dinner work for your family, finding a synagogue you want to be a part of and preparing your home—not only the physical space, but the loving values you want to embrace with those who are part of it.

Judaism offers some opportunities (both physical and emotional) to prepare your mind and heart for the arrival of the baby during these nine long months of waiting. While Jewish women generally shy away from the American nesting trends (like baby showers, designing the nursery, etc.) because of superstitious reasons, Jewish women can still find an outlet for all that pent-up *when-will-this-*

baby-arrive! energy.

As you're preparing your heart and home for motherhood, here are some especially Jewish things you can do:

Immerse in the mikvah

It can be both a spiritually uplifting and mindful practice to immerse in the mikvah. It's especially auspicious to do so in the ninth month of pregnancy, though there's no set date for when that should occur. There is no specific blessing to recite, but it is common to say a personal prayer for a healthy baby and for God to watch over you during labor and to help you with an easy and complete recovery. Check out the section *What is a mikvah?* in Chapter 4 for more details on what to expect!

Make changes to your routine

One of the first major changes to Jewish observance when you're pregnant is that you are no longer required to fast on days like Yom Kippur and Tisha B'Av. It is customary for a pregnant woman to avoid fasting even though Jewish people are commanded to do so on these days. That being said, while a pregnant woman doesn't need to fast she also doesn't need to feast. It's customary to have smaller meals, to wait perhaps a little longer than one normally would, just to feel a tinge of that same hunger sensation to have fulfilled the mitzvah. But the highest mitzvah is to care for yourself and to bring the baby safely into this world, so it is forbidden to put yourself in danger when pregnant (which fasting can do). As my mom would say, "There's nothing to be gained by it," and no prize to be given out for attempting to! Some Jewish women do request permission from their doctor to fast because they feel they are physically able to and that is fine as well; I personally am not one of those women!

Put another bun in the oven: Bake a challah (or a birth-day cake)

There are many old wives' tales about baking in the late stages of pregnancy, and the *bun in the oven* comparison is apropos. In the secular world, I've heard of the tradition to bake a birthday cake for your baby to encourage them to make their way out and celebrate with you. In Judaism there's a tradition to bake challah. Baking challah at any time in a woman's life is an especially holy act, and is considered part of her covenant with God—as it's one of the few obligations that are specifically commanded for women to perform (along with lighting Shabbat candles and going to the mikvah).

When a woman bakes challah it is said that she can communicate with the divine. Often, when she is braiding the dough, she will think about the prayers in her heart and ask God for His help. These days you can even see religious women posting on Instagram, letting others know that they will be baking challah and to send them names for those who need prayers. The mitzvah of separating the challah is also very closely associated with prayers for women, especially asking God for a soulmate and a child. The physical act of braiding challah is a means of connecting your *neshamah* (soul) to God.

The mitzvah of making challah is first mentioned in the Torah in the story of Sarah and her long struggle to conceive a child. When Abraham heard he would be visited by guests (who turned out to be angels of God), he prepared his home and a meal for them. He left the mitzvah of challah baking to his wife Sarah, who would later find out she was going to have a son.

There are even special types of challah, like the *shlissel* challah, which is baked into the shape of a key on the first Shabbat after Passover. It is said to be especially lucky to bake and eat a *shlissel* challah because it brings fortune to those who do.

The physical act of preparing the dough, kneading it, separating out the strands and braiding them back together can be a very spiritual and meditative practice. It's meant to take time and to be a special, even holy, food.

I have loved baking challah for years and there have been times, if I'm being honest, that the little braided beauties have totally flopped on me. They've turned out hard as rocks or I've missed ingredients along the way and they've been inedible. But I'm pretty sure they're teaching me a lesson in patience and humility. So take what you will from your own challah baking experiences; making a delicious challah is a culinary thrill like none other! And if you're not the type to bake your own, go out and buy some chocolate chip, raisin, seeded, rye...however you like it, enjoy!

Special honors in your synagogue

There are special honors in the synagogue for a couple expecting a baby. Some synagogues have a custom for the father to open the ark before the Torah reading during the mother's last month of pregnancy. It's a symbolic gesture to ask God to help open her womb for the baby to come to this world in safety and health. Ask your rabbi about having a special honor like opening the ark (*aron hakodesh*) or having an aliyah to the Torah in your final months of pregnancy. As explained by Chabad in their Life Cycle Mitzvot article on pregnancy, the Zohar says, "When the congregation takes out the Torah Scroll, the Heavenly Gates of Mercy are opened, and G-d's love is aroused."

As labor and delivery draw nearer, it's appropriate to ask God for protection and healing during this time. As with all things in the mystical and prayer world, it's important to give your *kavanah* (intention) to this experience, not so the prayers will work for God, but so they will work for you, as a way to pause and be mindful in your intent.

Give tzedakah

Giving to charity and performing deeds of loving kindness are an integral part of all major Jewish milestones. When there is a birth or bar mitzvah, family and friends often give to charity in lieu of or in addition to a present. This is a core part of Jewish values: to spend our time on Earth taking care of all of God's creatures and helping to repair this broken world. Aside from the *good luck* component of charity during pregnancy, doing *tzedakah* with your husband can be a meaningful and fun activity for the two of you to bond in a new way before your new arrival. Volunteering together can be an experience to take your mind off personal stresses and work on a project together. Another way to think about it is that you're setting up a way of life you'd like to continue as your family grows. Consider finding a place to volunteer your time as a family, where you can include your child.

It is especially auspicious to do *mitzvot* and acts of loving kindness before the baby arrives. Rebbe Nachman teaches that new beginnings are always difficult, but the practice of giving tzedakah opens our hearts and souls to new things. He compares *mitzvot* themselves to birth, likening contractions to the act of giving—because we never know how long it will take before our task is complete. He also recommends that this charity has to be done with intention and prayer; that these converge to speak to God. This can also be good practice in one of the most significant aspects of being a parent: giving selflessly.

Making Shabbat count

If you're looking for a way to mark the passage of time as each week goes by, hosting special Shabbat dinners can be a really enjoyable way to do so. Whether it's just you and your partner or you invite your friends (because, let's be honest, having a long evening to socialize will be a lot harder with a newborn!), you can take time as you light the candles each week to think about how far along you are and what's to come in the next week. During my later months of pregnancy I would often turn to my husband and son and say, "How many more Shabbats do you think we'll celebrate as just a family of three?" and everyone would guess.

These can also be a really beautiful stay-in date-nights where you put your phones and obligations down for a few hours and just enjoy time together. Some moms told me that they tried out different cookbook recipes during this time or had theme nights from different parts of the world to make it more fun and more of a culinary challenge. By setting aside Friday nights to spend together, these moms say they ended up creating a really nice space to just talk and be together as a couple in the chaos of preparing for parenthood.

One of the mothers I spoke with, Daniella, shared that she and her husband set out on a cookbook culinary journey and tried out one new recipe from the book each Shabbat during her pregnancy. It was fun to plan out the meals and to mark time in this way together.

Feed your body, nourish your soul

Having a kosher (or kosher-style) diet can be very beneficial to mom and baby and not just for spiritual reasons. Many of the *kashrut* customs are based on healthy clean eating. The way animal products are kashered is a detailed process ensuring they are free of bacteria and disease. Foods that are marked kosher on the packaging (with a *hechsher* or official sign-off from a kashering agency) have to meet high standards to receive this special rating. Also, eating kosher food will help you avoid some of the foods that can typically make pregnant women sick, like shellfish and sushi!

Kashrut is also about connecting body and soul, and pregnancy is a focused time in one's life where this connection is most vividly experienced. Thinking more about what you put into your body—because it is, in a sense, the first nutrition your baby is receiving—is a first act of taking care of your future child. Sure, you'd like a bacon double cheeseburger from McDonalds, but is now the best time in your life to have it?

Est Gezunterheyt! (as they say in Yiddish)—Eat in Good Health!

We've covered the scientific and the spiritual ways to prepare for motherhood. Let's move on to the sensational: Jewish food. Here's a Top 10 List ranked here, by me, as the best and most delicious options for pregnancy.

#1 Challah: Warm and fresh out of the oven is how I prefer it. Aside from being delicious, pleasing to even the pickiest of taste buds, and bland enough for even the worst of first trimesters, challah also has a spiritual component, as explained earlier in this chapter.

#2 Bagels: Similar to challah, but a little further from God and closer to Manhattan, lies the bagel. Another crowd pleaser for the first trimester to calm a weak stomach, bagels can be a warm welcome treat toasted up late at night when cravings can kick in.

#3 Kugels: Noodle, lokshen, bread, potato—you name it, I've eaten and loved it. Kugels are great for pregnancy because they come in both sweet and savory varieties and store well in the fridge and freezer. This makes them excellent homemade gifts for pregnant women or for after the baby is born.

#4 Friday Night Chicken: Can we talk about good old fashioned comfort food? OK. Chapter one, my bubbe's chicken. Cooked to perfection, falling-off-the-bone chicken and Friday nights just belong together. Chicken has good protein and most traditional roast chicken recipes involve putting chicken in a pan, sprinkling some spices on it and putting it into the oven. As *Barefoot Contessa* host Ina Garten would say, "How easy is that?!"

#5 Matzo Ball Soup: While we're on the subject of comfort food—I lived on my mother-in-law's matzo ball chicken soup during my first trimester of pregnancy. One of the really amazing added benefits is that a broth-based soup is a really easy way of taking in additional liquid, which I really struggled with. I could drink two bowls of chicken soup much more easily than two cups of water, and these soups have lots of great nutrients when made with fresh vegetables—and, of course—at least a cup-and-a-half of **love**.

#6 Brisket: Brisket is an easy way to get safe meat that's been well cooked and well-seasoned. Pregnancy is not the time to take chances with a rare cut of steak or burger, but go forth and brisket!

#7 Pickles: The sourness of these bingeable delicacies is what sets them apart for the pregnant palette, and at practically zero calories you can't go wrong. Just watch your sodium intake, because bloating is uncomfortable.

#8 Mandel Bread, Hamentashen, Rugelach, Babkah: Sure, Jewish desserts are a Sinai Desert away from healthy, but they're a lot less rich than classic American desserts like double-double chocolate sinful devils food whatnot, etc. Jewish desserts also tend to hold up really well in the fridge and freezer, so they're great for new moms and pregnant moms-to-be who don't have time or energy bake.

#9 Matzah: Part of me hates to even add this to the list because, oh-my-gosh, it is not my favorite. But if you're looking for a bland alternative to crackers in the first trimester, this can work. Do be cautious though: matzah can be very constipating and many pregnant women have issues with this in pregnancy!

#10 Dates: From the holy land of Eretz Yisrael if you can find them! Dates, if eaten daily, are supposed to help with labor because they share similar attributes to oxytocin. Talk to your doctor first before embarking on a pre-labor date regimen!

Foods to best to be cautious of or avoid

- **Manischewitz**: You're going to have stop guzzling that kiddush wine when you're pregnant, but one sip during the Shabbat kiddush is just fine!
- **Lox**: Of course this was about the only craving I had during pregnancy, even though I couldn't care less about it during the rest of my life. Smoked salmon can carry salmonella, which can transfer to the fetus, so it's best to avoid it.
- **Deli meat**: Another deli counter favorite that's best to avoid during pregnancy. Like lox, it can contain salmonella and listeria, which has even been linked to miscarriage.

I got a message from one of my YouTube followers asking if she was *really* craving something that wasn't kosher, could she eat it because she was pregnant? This really made me laugh: first, because I had never heard anything like it; and second, because I could totally see this scenario in cartoon form. God would be sitting in a fluffy cloud saying something like "Well...she **is** pregnant! Oy! Let her have the bacon!" *LOL*! If you're wondering the same thing the simple answer is no, there's no pregnancy excuse to eat something that isn't kosher. But cravings can be nearly impossible to ignore. So, if in your heart you have a reason that you must break *kashrut*, I won't be the one to stop you. If you're seriously struggling and *kashrut* is important to you, do talk to your rabbi!

8.
What to Expect from Everyone Else

The blessing of a Jewish community for parenting

Jewish communities are designed around supporting individual families. If you've heard that it takes a village to raise a child—this is the village. If you don't belong to a synagogue or aren't actively involved in a Jewish community, you might find that when you start having kids you would really welcome the resources a Jewish community can provide.

Do you have a friend who is having a baby around the same time that you are? If you do, that is amazing and such a gift! It is absolutely not true that you need to give up all your friends who aren't in the same stage of life as you are; but it does get a lot harder to make plans with them. On maternity leave, for example, it's really nice to have another mom to go on a walk with and complain about how little sleep you're getting. Not every friend has to be a friend for life; but women who share the same life situation as you are invaluable, and the Jewish community can be the perfect first stop for finding other women to connect with.

A lot of women I spoke to in researching this book list community as the single most important reason why they want to raise their kids within the Jewish faith. They spoke about a shared value system and a way of life that binds them to their Jewish friends and family. Of course it's important to have diversity in one's life and friend group, but I want to talk about how to find a Jewish community when you're pregnant or a new mom. A supportive Jewish community, whether it's connected to a synagogue, a community center, or even just a baby class can be so helpful to new moms!

Many Jewish couples are unaffiliated with official Jewish life before they get married and many still are when they're having their first child. They've left their hometowns and home-schuls and haven't yet felt the need to join a new synagogue. Having a child is a common time to seek out a Jewish community. Synagogues and community centers offer baby classes, playgroups or "Tot Shabbat" experiences geared toward little ones. Many of these gatherings are some of the first opportunities you'll have as a new parent to make friends with other families who are experiencing the same stage of life as you are.

How to find a synagogue that's right for you!

You don't need to become a synagogue member right at the beginning. Many synagogues and community centers offer their programs and classes for young kids for a small fee and most Shabbat playgroups or song sessions are free. It helps to look on Google Maps as your first option; finding a community close to you may provide the best circumstance for staying active and involved. Almost all synagogues in the U.S. have a website, and an internet search can let you get a look at a temple before you visit. Jewish nursery schools are also often housed in synagogues, too; so if this is something you are considering for the future, you may want to start your synagogue search from that direction.

Once you've narrowed down your list geographically try out some of the classes or services offered there to get a sense of the people and community. The best way to really narrow down your options is to experience them in person. You can go to any synagogue on a Saturday morning and get the feel for how they celebrate Shabbat, and what the personality of the congregation and rabbi are like. I like to take note of the age of the congregation and how they accommodate young families. In a large city with a large Jewish population (here's looking at you, LA!) there will be many options, so look for ones that offer things like "Tot Shabbats" or services geared toward preschool age children.

Connecting with the rabbi is also an important component of finding a synagogue that you feel comfortable in. Does his or her sermon move and inspire you? Does he or she have a welcoming attitude? Remember that this person will likely be involved in important life events for you, like a baby naming or bat mitzvah; so finding someone who makes these events more meaningful to you is important. A rabbi can also be a major source of emotional support to your family as you navigate a new life raising children.

And don't be discouraged! Many synagogues may not be a good fit, and some can feel totally uncomfortable when you first visit them. Finding a spiritual home can be like finding any other; it takes time and research to figure out what you really want and what's actually out there to fit your needs. If a traditional synagogue just feels wrong to you, there are lots of small new communities with different ways of bringing Jewish folks together. You can find services on the beach led by members of the community rather than a rabbi; you can find small gatherings in people's homes; or you can find larger congregations with various social groups like sisterhoods, youth groups and a Jewish day school on site. There are also communities that focus on *tikkun olam* (repairing the world) and social action.

If you're looking for an alternative to a big synagogue try Instagram as a search option. Look for tags like #jewishlife or #challahbake (which is used during community wide challah baking events) to find what people in your area are up to. If there are Jewish Instagrammers and social media influencers in your area, DM them and ask them to share their recommendations. You can also search a synagogue on Instagram to see what their events look like and if people tag them. Facebook is another excellent resource for local connections. Ask your community of friends for recommendations for local Shabbat classes and there will often be other moms who have been through this and found the best ones in the area.

Which community to join:
Orthodox, Conservative, Reform, Reconstructionist?

If you are new to Judaism or grew up without belonging to a synagogue, you may be faced with the choice of which denomination to choose for the first time. Many couples also face this dilemma if they are now at a different level of religious observance than how they grew up, or one partner doesn't feel comfortable in the other partner's denomination.

Even within each movement you will find different traditions and levels of observance, so this can be a difficult process. A very general guide is that Orthodox communities are the most observant according to traditional Jewish law or *halachah*, while Reform communities have adapted these traditions to most fit modern-day American life. However, there are members of any community who observe different customs and have their own level of observance.

If your goal is to find a welcoming community for new or growing families, start by finding a synagogue that offers the facilities and opportunities you need, like a nursery school or Shabbat playgroups. Then really consider what type of community you want to be a part of. Many religious communities, like Chabad (a global Orthodox synagogue network) are very welcoming of families who may not have a particularly religious background but want to learn more. However, if you have a liberal outlook and female members of your family who want to play an active role in services or become bat mitzvah, then starting at an Orthodox schul will not be a good fit.

The community you already know and sorta kinda love:
your extended family

You might think you're the one having the baby, but a lot of other family members are probably feeling pretty involved, too. Judaism is very much a family-centered religion and it's a rare Jewish family that doesn't have some extended members eager to share an opinion about a new baby's arrival. Jewish tradition involves and includes family members from the beginning by giving them special honors at the baby's bris or baby naming, and Jewish holidays and life cycle events are very much centered around the family. So it makes sense to start thinking about extended family members during your pregnancy months. And of course there is your partner: as the father of the baby, he's got a 50% genetic stake in what's about to happen and may have more than 50% of the opinions on how things should or shouldn't go.

As we're halfway through the book, it's time to really dive into a topic most Jewish women might prefer to avoid: your mother-in-law! I've shared a video on my YouTube channel all about these crazy creatures and how I actually love and am good friends with mine. So I speak from experience when I say that they're not all that bad! It really is a very negative stereotype in American culture that all mothers-in-law are pushy and annoying; but there is some truth to the idea that when you get married you aren't just marrying your partner, but his whole family as well.

During sessions with our rabbi before he officiated our wedding ceremony, Rabbi Ed Feinstein, Senior Rabbi of Valley Beth Shalom in Encino, California, would say that every marriage is an intermarriage. In one way or another you're blending two families, and it isn't always a harmonious union.

If you do have a positive relationship with your in-laws, and your mother-in-law in particular, then having a baby will likely be a time of continued closeness and shared happiness. If she lives close by she will likely be supportive and helpful, run errands, be able and willing to babysit, and just generally be a source of comfort in your new life as parents. But if you, like many, many women out there, fear/loathe/annoy/are annoyed by your mother in law, then bringing a baby into the family may exacerbate these issues.

If you're already sensing conflict on the horizon, the most important thing is that you and your partner are united in your decisions. This can be a good time to talk to a counselor or couples therapist if extended family conflict is infiltrating your relationship. Pregnancy can be a time of heightened emotions and vulnerability, and you may find yourself arguing with your partner more than you had before. Jewish tradition puts family first. Having open dialogue and communication between you and your partner will really help even before the baby arrives.

The generations and opinions are adding up!

One important thing to keep in mind when dealing with your parents (or your partner's parents) and a newborn is that a lot of advice and knowledge from when you were little is outdated today. It's a changing world; but many of our moms and mothers-in-law are of the opinion that they successfully raised you and your siblings, so they know how to do things best. Even if they are up to date on car seat standards and sleeping guidelines, this is still your time to assert yourself as a parent and not fall victim to self-doubt from someone who has done it all before.

Here are some typical things that the previous generation believed:

- The sun is a cure for jaundice in the first days of life: MYTH. Jaundice can indicate that your newborn isn't getting enough breast-milk in his first days of life. It's critical to have his levels measured—especially if he's exclusively breastfed and is looking jaundiced.
- Babies should sleep on their stomachs: MYTH. Newborns should sleep on their backs.
- Don't let the baby nap too long in the day—she won't sleep at night: MYTH. Aside from day/night confusion, generally sleep begets sleep—and a well-rested baby is a happy, sleepy baby! An overtired baby can be really difficult to get to sleep at night.
- Don't give the baby peanut butter: MYTH. check the American Academy of Pediatrics guidelines on introducing solid foods. They have updated their recommendations to testing peanut butter early

(around 5 months) to avoid allergies.

- Don't spoil the baby with cuddles and holding them: MYTH. This is one of my personal favorites. Say it with me, folks: BABIES CANNOT BE SPOILED!
- Don't feed them at night: MYTH. Some babies need to be fed at night. Newborns need to eat every few hours, and even older babies may require the nutrition; so ask your pediatrician first!
- Don't breastfeed too long: MYTH. New science shows the benefit of breastfeeding through one year and beyond!
- Get a babysitter: MYTH. Well, maybe not a myth; but it's up to **you** to decide when you want to leave your baby in someone else's care and who that person should be!

So how to handle this unwanted advice? Be kind, be cautious, and be careful!

Be kind to those who are offering advice. People don't think about or give opinions about things they don't care about. Just because they are wrong or annoying doesn't mean they aren't trying to be helpful. So, appreciate that someone out there loves your child enough to have an opinion about how they're cared for.

Be cautious. Don't just dismiss everything they say or put up boundaries about what is and isn't on the table to discuss. You don't want to alienate family members who can be helpful with newborn care.

Be careful. Remember that many parents have hazy memories of the early years of motherhood (I mean, who can even remember what they had for breakfast yesterday, let alone their son's nap schedule from 30 years ago). And they may be quite adamant that they did it a certain way and it worked for them, so be careful of this logic pattern—"*Well, all my babies had bumpers on their crib and none of them suffocated.*" That fact doesn't mean that crib bumpers aren't dangerous and suffocation hazards; it just means not every baby (including yourself or your husband) died because they were placed in a crib with bumpers.

I guess it comes down to this: advice is like food in the break room. It's usually old, it's often not that great, but if you never take a look at it you might miss a free chocolate cupcake!

Let's talk about Dad

Are you feeling like since you got pregnant your partner is just **doing everything wrong**?! If so, you're not alone. Thanks to a gnarly combination of pregnancy hormones, exhaustion, and general unease, it's really common for women to feel distant and easily frustrated by their partners. After all, they got to participate in the fun part of making the baby, and now you're the one doing all the hard work. It can be difficult come to grips with a really draining first trimester or uncomfortable pregnancy symptoms when nothing changes for him.

Almost all the women I interviewed for this book shared funny stories (or maybe funny now, but not at the time) about how their partners just "didn't get it." Partners tend to say the wrong things, buy the wrong things at the store, and just generally frustrate you. I know from personal experience; my husband frustrated me just by the fact that he could go on living his day to day life without a giant bump preventing him from tying his shoes—it just isn't fair!

Of course they are very likely still the loving husbands you married, but this is a big learning curve for them as well. Try to exercise some kindness, compassion, and patience for them and consider whether you're unfairly taking out your irritability on them. Judaism places the relationship between partners very highly and stresses the importance of working on communication and preserving the marital relationship. Do you have an effective strategy for talking these things through? Is your partner really not supporting you, helping you and caring for you at this time? If you're having to pause or have legitimate concerns, then now is the time to seek help and counseling if dealing with these issues between just the two of you isn't working.

Your partner may also be feeling his own apprehension and anxiety about what bringing a new baby into this world may bring and how his life is going to change. In a way, women have more time to prepare because our bodies are constantly reminding us that something is changing; whereas it can all feel a bit more sudden for guys.

In our home (even though my husband might not readily admit to this), I think it was hard for him in those first few weeks after we brought our son home from the hospital for him to go back to work. He knew how much he was needed at home and also how lovely and enjoyable those early days were. I had a much longer maternity leave than him and the sacrifice that he made each day missing out on time with his new son to go to work really hit me. I tried to show my appreciation and love for him by saying goodbye each morning with my son with something like "Thank you for going to work today, Dada, so that we could stay home. We love you!" We also implemented a date night every week. On date night we didn't actually leave the house because, well, having a non-sleeping newborn meant no energy for things like Uber, reservations, etc. So instead we used this night as a night off chores and work: no dishes, no emails, just yummy take-out food and TV. Of course, feel free to make that more romantic if you're so inclined, but this is what worked for us.

I asked my husband Andrew what his advice for first-time dads is and this is what he said: "Make silly faces and bounce on a ball." This advice makes me smile because it's so simple—but it also really does work. Before our son was born my husband would say he wasn't good with babies. He knew he was great with toddlers and little kids; he loves to play and run around and make mayhem and was always the one with all four of our nephews climbing on top of him. As our son now is two years old it's no surprise my husband was right: the best part of our son's day is when Dad's car pulls into the driveway after work.

However, my husband learned that he actually was good with babies too because he trusted his own instincts. He learned how to bounce on an exercise ball to calm a crying baby and he used his natural ability to be silly and make others smile to keep our little one calm and entertained. He also added, "Don't sweat the small stuff. They're much more resilient than you think." Babies seem incredibly delicate when they are first born and I've seen many fathers step tenderly (awkwardly) into those first days of holding and changing a newborn, but they get the hang of it soon enough!

He said that he tells expecting dads to let the mom lay out the basic schedule and what she wants for the baby (in other words, listen to Mom), but also feel confident to take charge and make some decisions on your own. It's a delicate balance and at the beginning and there's only so much you can do, especially if mom is breastfeeding. But he says, "Make sure to find something you can do, and spend as much time as you can with the baby." Bonding is important for Dad, too!

If your partner is looking for some inspiration on being a Jewish dad, here's some quick info for him:

Our ancient rabbis taught that a father has four major obligations: to circumcise his son; to teach him Torah; to help find him a wife; and to teach him a way to earn money. These are stated in the Talmud and there's even an additional commentary that the father should also teach his child to swim. What can we take away from these very specific requirements? That to be a good Jewish dad, a father must enable his children to lead a life of their own. To help them grow up and be able to learn, provide for a family and create a family of their own. And swimming is great, too—because kids are better off knowing how to swim before they head for summer camp, and pools can be dangerous places if you don't know how to swim.

"Train a child in the way that he should go" (Proverbs 22:6).

It might be a really interesting conversation to ask your partner about their own father, and to share your experience as well. What was their dad's role in the family? Did he work outside the home and contribute equally to childcare (or not?) and how has that influenced your own expectations of fatherhood. Then in terms of Jewish life, did dad share in the same Jewish values as mom and what did that mean in terms of who went to synagogue and how holidays were observed. By looking back at your own upbringing you may more clearly see what works and didn't work in your mind.

Creating an Ethical Will

It's a good idea to create a legal will when you have a baby and to think about who will take care of your future children and how your financial assets should be distributed in the event that one or both parents pass away. In Jewish tradition, there's also a custom of creating what's called an Ethical Will. These documents, called *tzava'ot* in Hebrew, expand on the legal provisions a traditional will would cover and can give more insight into how they would like their heirs to live once they have died. In many ways the ethical will is a distribution of the wealth of wisdom that people have, as opposed to their material possessions.

Rabbi Myrna Matsa spoke to me about how she talks to Jewish couples about creating a different type of ethical will, one for their children to open at the age of 21. Traditionally ethical wills are created when one is near the end of their life or facing sickness, but Rabbi Matsa shared with me that there are other ways to use this type of document. Rabbi Matsa counsels couples who are preparing for parenthood and who come to her with anxiety over how to raise their children Jewishly and with the Jewish values that are important to them. She helps couples write out a document that details exactly what these values, hopes and dreams are for these children.

This exercise allows couples the time and place to focus their attention on these critically important but often neglected discussions. Then the letter is tucked safely away until the child becomes a legal adult, and then is given to them as a gift. You can create your own letter or ethical will for your baby as an exercise with your partner to help you both focus on what are the important attributes and qualities you want to pass along to your child. You could even update it as they grow with stories and memories of their Jewish experiences along the way. It could be an especially meaningful bar-mitzvah or graduation gift as well if you so choose.

9.
Jewish Baby Names.
Jewish Names, Hebrew Names
and How to Choose.

Why are names so important in Judaism?

Judaism has a thing with names—God's name especially. God is so holy, so deserving of reverence, that we should never utter His true name. Even those in the Bible to whom God revealed his name were not able to say it aloud because it cannot be pronounced. We have dozens of ways to refer to God, each name with its own inherent nuanced meaning. So naturally, Judaism has a thing about names—and it is clear in many *midrash* stories and throughout Jewish traditions that names are meaningful.

Some of the most significant stories in the Torah are all about names. When Abraham and Sarah become the very first Jewish people their names are changed from Avram and Sarai. When Jacob wrestles with an angel of God in a dream he is then given the name Israel. When Queen Esther's story begins in the Megillah reading on Purim she is known by her Jewish name, Hadassah.

In Jewish tradition names can carry a person's entire history and identity. In ancient times, people did not have surnames as we do now. A person was given their first name and were then referred to as *ben* (son of) So-and-so for a boy or Bat (daughter of) So-and-so for a girl. For example, a boy named David with a father named Saul would be called David ben Saul. Who you are is where you came from—it's all in the name.

How Jewish English and Hebrew names are chosen

I've always said picking a baby name is easy; it's agreeing on one with your partner that's tough. At this point in your life you've probably been forced to eliminate about 90% of all popular baby names because someone close to you has already taken it for their child, or you know someone who has the name and you don't like them (just me?). Once you have picked out a name you actually do like, you then need to find something that works well with the baby's last name. By the time you have your list and cross-reference it with your partner's, you may be left with nothing!

If, on the other hand, you are overwhelmed with options, giving your child a Jewish name can make the process a little easier. Jewish children are traditionally given two names: an English name and a Hebrew name. Sometimes this can be the same name; when a child's English name is a Biblical name, Yiddish name, or Hebrew name, parents can use the same name for both. The name Gideon, for example, is Gideon in both Hebrew and English. Some couples choose the Hebrew translation of an English name for the Hebrew name: for example, a girl named Rose might be given the Hebrew name *Shoshanah*, which means rose in Hebrew. Or a couple may find a Hebrew version of an English name: for example, Samuel would be *Shmuel* in Hebrew. The child's Hebrew name will be used in Hebrew school and whenever they are called to the Torah in synagogue, such as on their bar or bat mitzvah. It also will be the name used on their marriage contract, the *ketubah*, when they get married.

While choosing the right Hebrew name can take time, giving your child more than one name can provide an opportunity for each parent to have a say in the naming decision. Hebrew names also offer another opportunity to add meaning to your baby's name. You can pick a character from the Bible whose story you admire—although you should really do your research on that one. Some of our Biblical ancestors have histories that would raise eyebrows by today's standards!

Traditionally, Ashkenazi Jewish families name babies (either their English or Hebrew names, or often both) after someone who has passed away. This is an enormous honor to bestow, and I can't think of anything that quite compares to it. It's a spiritual connection to the generations that came before, and a prayer for who the child will hopefully grow to emulate. So it's important that you have loving memories of the person if you choose to use their name (or a version of their name), and hope that your child will share some of their positive attributes.

It's common to use just the first letter or first few letters of the relative's name when choosing a name for your child. For example, my son Max is named after both of his great-grandfathers: Montague and Mayer. Other popular examples include Abe to Andrew, Morris to Michael, and Saul to Sam—as many Jewish couples today want to give their children modern names that still honor the more Yiddish-sounding traditional ones previous generations held. Among Sephardic families, the tradition is to name children after their grandparents even if they are still alive. The first child is usually named after their father's parent, and the next child after the mother's parent.

It is also a beautiful custom to choose a character from the Torah portion that corresponds to the baby's birth; or if a Jewish holiday coincides with the baby's birth, you could choose a name from that story.

One of the mothers I spoke with shared that she faced a difficult choice when it came to honoring a family member who had passed away after struggling with drug and alcohol abuse. On the one hand, she loved this relative and wanted to help keep their memory a blessing; on the other hand, the sting of the end their life was still too raw. If you are struggling with honoring someone with a similar situation in your family, I encourage you to talk to your rabbi about it, but also follow your own heart on this.

Some Jewish families choose to only use this custom of honoring relatives for a child's Hebrew name and choose the English name separately. Or they might choose not to honor a relative at all and just choose a name that has meaning to them.

I am lucky enough to have a healthy and happy baby boy, but before he was born I lost a pregnancy at five months. To honor that loss, we gave our son the middle name Seth. In the Torah, after Eve's son Abel is killed she prays for God to help her with this loss, and Seth is given to her. For our family, this name is a way to thank God for the gift of a healthy baby boy after losing one so precious to us.

In researching this book, I asked a lot of Jewish mothers how they picked their children's names. Here are some of the most creative ideas I heard!

Rachel (children aged 3, 6, 9) chose her children's names based on who she and her husband wanted to honor in the family. Then using that same first letter, they looked for names that would be the same in Hebrew and English, which is a beautiful tradition!

Shira (children aged 1, 4, 6) said she felt her children's Hebrew names were their first connection to Judaism, so she chose Hebrew names like the one she was given (Shira means song in Hebrew) for them as their English names as well.

Miranda Kemp (Instagram handle @Mirandahkemp), whose children are 3 and 1, said that for her, baby naming was not "traditionally Jewish" and instead chose to give her boys their grandfathers' names as their middle names and then to honor her husband's Scottish heritage in her sons' first names.

Looking for inspiration?

Each year the website *Kveller.com* puts out a few different lists of Jewish baby names—unique ones, popular ones, etc. They are a great resource if you're looking for some ideas they include the meanings and explanations of the names. Over the course of the past decade, these names have made the list of *Kveller.com*'s "most popular" Jewish baby names:

GIRLS

Abigail	Eliana	Ellie
Anna	Eliza	Hannah
Ava	Elizabeth	Lilah
Charlotte	Ella	Sadie

BOYS

Alexander	Ethan	Matthew
Asher	Ezra	Michael
Benjamin	Gabriel	Nathan
Caleb	Isaac	Noah
Daniel	Jacob	Samuel
David	Joshua	Simon
Elijah	Levi	

Here's a list of Jewish and Hebrew names (and their meanings) popular over the past decade as listed on several baby name websites:

GIRLS

Adina: delicate

Ayala: gazelle or doe

Esther: Purim's queen

Hannah: favor or grace

Leah: delicate; one of the Torah's matriarchs

Miriam: Moses's sister

Naomi: pleasantness

Noa: movement

Rivka: (Rebecca) Matriarch in the Bible

Sarah: Princess and Abraham's wife

Shira: song

Shoshana: rose

Talia: dew

Tamar: palm tree

Yael: female prophet

Zara: seed

Ziva: radiance, of God's light

BOYS

Alon: oak tree

Ariel: lion

Asher: blessed

Daniel: God is my judge

David: King David, beloved

Eitan: strong

Ezra: help

Joseph: to increase

Levi: ancestor of one of the 12
  tribes, priestly class

Meir: one who shines

Noah: rest and comfort

Noam: tenderness

Raviv: rain

Uri: my light

When to announce the name for a boy?

There is a lot of Jewish superstition surrounding a baby's name and it is rare for Jewish families to share the name they are choosing until the baby is born. When a boy is born, it is tradition not to say his name until his bris, eight days later. The baby boy's name is not technically received until his bris, just as Abraham's name was changed (from Avram) when he had his own bris (at 99!). According to the ancient Zohar text, it is at the bris that the "full measure of his soul" is received; and accordingly, he cannot be truly named until that happens. In ultra-Orthodox circles families observe a *vach nacht*, where they stay up all night before the bris praying, reciting portions of the Torah, and saying the *shema* prayer in order to protect the baby before his name is bestowed upon him the next day.

It is because Jewish baby names hold such meaning and importance, and because they are the connection between the body (the physical world) and the soul (the metaphysical), that announcing the name for the first time at the bris elevates the holiness of the ceremony. In my family, we struggled with the decision of when to announce our son's name. We had a lot of pressure from family members to let them know what it was beforehand, but we really wanted to wait to reveal it. On a practical level, I didn't like the idea that if we announced the name before our son's bris we'd essentially have 80 people over to our house to watch him be circumcised. I felt that by sharing his name and the meaning behind it at the bris, it put the focus of the day on that. In the end, I followed my heart and was happy that I did. Although we did quietly fill out his name on his birth certificate just before leaving the hospital, which is something I was told to do, because changing it after the fact in some states can be a hassle.

Many people find this custom entirely inconvenient (for instance, it's tough at the hospital when you're filling out forms and insurance information to say to the nursing staff that actually the baby does have a name but you can't share it yet). In some states you need to apply for a change to the birth certificate if you don't want to write the baby's name down when he's born, so there are practicalities of this decision to keep in mind. One easy compromise to consider is saving the announcement of just the baby's Hebrew name until the bris or naming ceremony.

One of the mothers I interviewed, Rachel (children aged 3,6,9), kept her son's name a secret until his bris, but because they had to use his real name at the pediatricians office, they arrived at his first appointment with some family in tow—who all heard the name the day before the bris when the nurse in the waiting room called them back! *Oy!*

One last thing to consider about timing: the earlier you announce the baby's name, the more you open your choice to opinion and advice from family and friends. You may think someone close to you might have good constructive criticism; but if you really love a name, one off-the-cuff comment can really sour a name for you. And in the end, everyone has an opinion. Pick a name you love and don't worry about what others think.

And for a girl?

The same traditions and superstitions about waiting a week after a baby girl is born to say her name don't apply. Many Jewish parents do prefer to wait the same eight days in the spirit of egalitarianism, while others choose to wait until the next Torah service (the Torah is read on Monday, Thursday and Saturday) to do so. Most commonly, a baby girl's name is shared when she is born.

It is now popular to have a naming ceremony for a girl (discussed more in Chapter 11), where her Hebrew name is shared and often her family is called up to the Torah and celebrated. These ceremonies are usually planned for at least a month or more after the baby is born, so parents may wait to share her Hebrew name until then.

A closing thought

Ultimately, there's very little you as a parent can control about who your child will become: their personality, their interests, their eye color. But their name is the one element of their identity you can give them with full intention and determination. What a blessing!

In Judaism, giving a name is giving a blessing. There are many connections in the Torah between the Jewish people and stars in the sky. Psalm 147 says that God so loved each individual star that he gave every one of them a name. So, as God showed His love for the stars by giving them each a name, we show our love for our children the same way.

10.

Having faith in an interfaith family

What to expect when one parent isn't Jewish

Before our wedding, Rabbi Ed Feinstein who officiated our ceremony, told my husband and me that every marriage is an intermarriage. In one way or another, when two people come together to create a family, they bring with them a whole lifetime's worth of customs, experiences and traditions that they need to fit together. My parents had season tickets to the Los Angeles Philharmonic; my husband's to the Washington Capitals hockey team. Sure, we were both raised in nice Jewish homes by nice Jewish parents, but there was still a lot of disconnect between what we believed and what we valued based on how we grew up. We didn't have to figure out the "December Dilemma" (Hanukkah or Christmas), but we did have a Sunday dilemma (football or, please God, anything else!) and we disagreed about how kosher to keep our home and how often we should attend synagogue.

For an interfaith couple, these differences can be magnified because of a whole entourage of family members who feel like there's a win/lose aspect to religious observance. There is a saying in Judaism that with each new baby the world begins anew, and that profound concept is especially true when it comes to the world of your family and traditions when your baby is born.

Rabbi Stutman explained to me that, "Religion is not always rational; it's primal." When a baby is born, those long-forgotten memories of one's own childhood can resurface. Things that didn't seem to matter when you were just a couple now take on a whole new level of significance when two become three. For example, a partner raised Christian may never attend church now, but may still feel uncomfortable not baptizing his baby if it's tradition in his family to do so.

Often the difficulties of an interfaith relationship arise in wedding planning: who will officiate, where will it take place, what customs will be incorporated; but once a couple makes it past this initial hurdle, the stress and family tension can dissipate for a while. When a couple is expecting a baby, this may be a time in their life when their decisions about religion come into question. Often this can come to the forefront when deciding on a bris or circumcision, because it occurs just days after the baby is born and can force the issue right away.

If the mother of the baby is not Jewish (Judaism is passed down matrilineally in most communities), a rabbi may require the mother to convert first. Or the bris can still occur on the eighth day and the baby will undergo a conversion ceremony including immersion in the *mikvah* (ritual bath) later. Having a baby naming for a girl allows more flexibility as it is a relatively new tradition; but again, the mother's religion and the issue of conversion may arise (see more about conversion in the next chapter).

One of the mothers I interviewed (Katie, who has a one-year-old son) said that being in an interfaith relationship was never an issue for her and her husband. Although they had many religious ties in terms of schools they attended and community organizations they were part of, they never considered themselves very religious. While she grew up in a Christian home, she had many Jewish friends; so Jewish culture didn't feel so foreign. They took the basics of each of their religions: the value of family, of being kind to others, and of sharing and taking care of those less fortunate—and then let the other aspects of religion fall away. Katie told me that "We have embraced each other's traditions"—like celebrating Christmas together, but keeping the focus on love and family.

Katie explained, "When we thought about how we would navigate having a baby, it really was about how to make sure that the grandparents felt like their cultures were being valued." That's when the decision between baptism and bris came up. Circumcision was something that made sense to her, but the traditional bris ceremony didn't. And that's where compromise came in—by including a blessing before the circumcision which took place in the hospital.

When it came to choosing a name for their son, they both gravitated toward Biblical names and ended up going with one. They wanted their son to have a strong name that meant something important to people of all faiths.

Katie had some very wise words about what it means to raise a child with both Jewish and Christian religions as a part of their history and identity. In reference to her son, she said, "I think it will be good for him to be raised with two religions. He will see that just because people don't believe the same things, doesn't mean they are better or worse than anyone else. Love is love and kindness is kindness—the stories from the Torah teach important lessons, and so do the stories from the New Testament ... I like the idea of giving my son options so that he can make up his own mind about what to believe and what to have faith in."

Rabbi Stutman reminded me that children have a tendency to believe the way they are being raised is normal. It might not be your experience to be raised with two faiths, but it will be their normal and their life. As the number of Jewish young adults who intermarry increases (as has been the growing trend for the past few decades), these families will continue to find more and more community members who share their experience.

That being said, it can be helpful to start the conversations of what this new normal will look like even before the baby is born. Does having a Hebrew school education or a bar mitzvah matter to you? Can you embrace Hanukkah and Christmas in December? Rather than arriving at these moments and making a decision "by default," Rabbi Stutman encourages couples she counsels to think about their priorities and invest in them. She is also a fan of specificity: one person's idea of what a holiday celebration or religious upbringing really looks like can differ greatly from their partner's. She also encourages families to find community, *kehila*. This is an essential component of Judaism and it's just as important (if not more so!) for interfaith families whose lives don't look like traditional Jewish families.

How to handle the grandparents

How you raise your child is, of course, a decision for you and your partner to make together. However, it may help to be sensitive to your own parents, who you want to be involved in your child's life. They are likely feeling powerless in the fate (and faith!) of their new grandchild and it can feel like a type of loss to them if you don't plan to raise the child in the same religion in which they raised you. It can help to talk to them about the decision, and let them know that choosing a different spiritual path doesn't mean you are choosing to be any less a part of their lives.

Among the women I interviewed from interfaith marriages, there were many humorous, loving and sometimes nightmare-inducing stories about how grandparents become involved in the religious upbringing of their grandchild. If you go to synagogue, you'll very often find that the grandparents are the ones bringing little ones to Tot Shabbat. And it's common to see grandparents signing kids up for Jewish activities or even Hebrew school. This trend is consistent with many grandparents being caregivers, now that it's so common for both parents to be working full time. When they have a choice, Jewish grandparents will frequently choose Jewish activities for their grandchildren. It can be helpful to think about these things before the baby arrives, and talk to grandparents about your feelings. Or you can take each of these events as they come if that works better for you.

Many synagogues and Jewish community centers also offer classes and support groups for interfaith families. If your parents are struggling, a quick online search for "interfaith grandparent classes" in your area may yield some helpful results. Aside from the material covered in these courses, which includes topics like how to have sensitive conversations and how to preserve your family traditions, it's also great for grandparents to find a supportive community of peers to talk to about these issues.

Fostering a spirit of inclusion and togetherness at a Jewish bris or baby naming

There is so much excitement, anticipation and emotion wrapped up in a baby's birth—and not just for the parents. Grandparents and siblings—who will play a significant role in the baby's life—also want to be included in the celebration of their birth.

Part of this inclusion can take place during the baby's naming ceremony or bris. Non-Jewish family members may feel uncomfortable having a formal role in a bris or baby naming because they don't want to make a mistake or do the wrong thing, and many are nervous they'll be asked to read Hebrew or say a prayer they don't know or aren't comfortable with. Family members may also be unaware of the ceremony altogether and may not know that there are opportunities for their involvement.

Talk to your rabbi about including non-Jewish relatives in the rituals by having them carry the baby, read a prayer, or stand by the parents during the ceremony. If your relatives aren't comfortable with what's happening, it might be best to talk to them about how they're feeling and let them know that having them involved in these special moments is important to you.

You can also consider adding non-Jewish traditions to a ceremony with decorations and important objects. Even including a grandmother's famous dessert recipe by serving her cookies to your guests is a thoughtful way to say "we are honoring your traditions" on this day. Couples can also use decorations to honor family traditions. For example, you could display framed photographs of family members from when they were born, or include an important color—like red for Chinese family members. Even a beloved childhood book on display from different members of the family can be a lovely way to include them.

If there will be non-Jewish guests in attendance at the bris or baby naming (which is very common), make sure your rabbi or mohel explains what's going on and includes a welcoming message to everyone at the start of things. It is also helpful for the non-Jewish parent to welcome their guests and make them feel comfortable with a short speech at the beginning. This can be an appropriate time to name the grandparents on both sides of the family and thank them for their love and for being there.

If you anticipate conflict with your in-laws, it may be best to discuss matters with them much ahead of the birth of the baby. After the baby arrives, everyone will be very tired and emotional (especially the new parents) and may say things they otherwise wouldn't. Also, if the conversation does get heated but happens months before the baby's arrival, this will give everyone some time to heal before the big day.

Nowadays it is becoming more common to create your own mixed-faith ceremony to welcome a baby, and many rabbis will help you create a ceremony that works for your family. Although rare, there are joint naming ceremonies—I even came across the term *bris-tism*!

The Third Trimester

Planning a bris or baby naming

What is a bris, and why is it so important to Jewish families?

Planning a bris can be an extremely stressful experience; hosting an event just days after you've given birth can be really hard. But before we get into the details of planning a bris, let's first talk about what's beautiful and lovely about the mitzvah of the *brit milah* ceremony.

A bris, or *brit milah* as it is known in Hebrew, is the religious circumcision ceremony for a Jewish baby boy. It is traditional for the ritual to be performed on the eighth day of the baby boy's life, unless the baby has medical issues which prevent it. Remember that days in Judaism begin at sunset; so if a baby is born at 10:00 pm on a Monday night, his first day of life is actually Tuesday according to the Jewish calendar. A baby born at Monday at 2pm would have his bris the following Monday, but a baby born on a Monday at 10pm (after sunset) would have his bris the following Tuesday.

Let's go over that again:

If your baby boy is born on **Monday BEFORE Sunset** then his bris is the next **Monday**.

If your baby boy is born on **Monday AFTER Sunset** then his bris is the next **Tuesday**.

There are many interpretations as to why the bris occurs on the eighth day. One take on it is that the first seven days of life represent the seven days that God took to create the physical world. On the eighth day we can begin to think about the spiritual world, which is what the bris is all about. Another is that it was customary to wait a few days after birth until the baby is strong enough to undergo the procedure.

A bris is such a special, holy and important event that it is even allowed to take place on Shabbat! A bris is traditionally performed by a *mohel*, someone who is trained in the religious and surgical procedure of the circumcision.

"Wait, did you say...bris or brit?" This is just a dialectic thing. The Hebrew letter *Tav* is often pronounced as an *s*.

The bris is one of the most significant events of Jewish life. The word *brit* means covenant, and the *brit milah* ceremony is the foundational connection between man and God. The first mention of the *brit milah* in the Torah is in the *L'chi Lach* reading: Abraham is commanded to circumcise himself to show his commitment to God, and in return God promises to make him a father to a great people (Genesis 17:10-14). The commandment of a bris is a ritualistic and symbolic expression of a parent's promise to continue Abraham's covenant, to obey God's commandments, and to raise their child within the Jewish faith.

A circumcision, to be clear and technical, is the surgical removal of the foreskin on the head of the penis. I'll save you some searching and let you know that WebMD suggests that two thirds of all baby boys in the United States are circumcised, and the main medical benefit of the procedure is better hygiene. There are various types of techniques used to perform this surgery, and different pain medications for the baby—more on that in the *What to ask a mohel* section.

It is normal to feel anxious about the bris!

OK, so it can be a lovely tradition, but let's take a second to get into which aspects of the experience are stressful for new moms. First, your baby boy (to whom you've only just given birth days before) has to undergo surgery in a sensitive area of his little body. This early in his life he's probably barely been held by anyone besides Mom, Dad, doctors and nurses—so putting him into a situation you have little control over can be really upsetting. Second, your newborn is having surgery performed on him, and often it's not in a medical setting. This can be really anxiety-inducing for some people. But you are not alone!

In past generations the mother didn't always attend the bris. Her baby was escorted to the ceremony by a relative and brought back to her afterwards. Personally, I did not want to be separated from my baby, so that did not appeal to me. But if you are too exhausted, in pain from birth, or just can't bring yourself to face all the people or the surgery itself then, *you don't need to go!*

Then there's what for me was the really scary part, so let's get this out of the way. The baby doesn't usually cry much during the procedure, but you're bound to have a cranky baby after it's done. Usually the mom will take the baby away from the celebration to nurse him, give him some pain medicine, and help him fall asleep. The excitement, number of people, and the commotion of it all in addition to feeling sore is a lot for a tiny baby. For me, this was the first time I really had to comfort my son—who up to that point had been a very quiet and sleepy newborn.

If you are a first-time mom, my best advice is to designate an experienced mom (maybe a close friend who has gone through this recently) to help you during this time. Most guests will know not to bother you at this time but it may also help to have someone stand by the door to your room to politely make sure well wishers give you the time you need to comfort and calm your baby.

It also helps to research some comforting techniques beforehand. For example, many babies like to be rocked or swung in their mama's arms; others just need to hear *shh, shh* white noise with gentle rocking until they fall asleep. For my son, the combination of the loud *shh* noise (we stood underneath a loud ceiling fan in our bathroom) and the rhythmic movement of me bouncing on an exercise ball while holding him worked. With a pediatrician-recommended dose of infant Tylenol and a nap, most babies are totally fine within a few hours.

So many women I interviewed for this book, who were raised in warm Jewish communities and who had traditional Jewish marriages, were still reluctant or even refused to have a traditional bris celebration for their son. Though they supported circumcision, they preferred to postpone a celebration until they were healed from birth. While I learned about all sorts of different experiences and celebrations, one thing was universal among these moms: whatever choice they made, each one of them had strong feelings about a bris.

One of the Jewish mothers I spoke to, Sandra (who is already a grandmother and whose children are now 32, 39 and 43 years old), had her first son in the 1970s. She remembers vividly how she had wanted to have a bris outside of the hospital, but was discouraged by her husband and mother to do so. They had just moved to a new neighborhood, weren't very religious and didn't know many people to invite. She still regrets her decision all these years later, because to her having a bris was such a crucial important Jewish custom.

My advice from hearing so many stories—both positive and negative—about the bris, is to just follow your own heart and try as best you can not to be influenced by what others say you should do. It will be an emotional and likely hard day for you even if it all goes beautifully according to plan, so try to think about setting it up in a way that will make it a bit easier and more enjoyable.

How to plan a bris... where to start?

Practically speaking, outside of the actual circumcision which the *mohel* will take care of, a bris involves planning a party much like any other. It is also customary to serve a meal, known as a *seuda*, after the bris ceremony. This tradition started back with Abraham who made a meal after circumcising his son Isaac.

The first decision as a new parent you'll need to make about a bris is whether or not to have one. If you do want to have your son circumcised but don't want to host a bris event to do so, you can have the procedure done in a hospital. Many Jewish families elect to have the procedure done in the hospital on the eighth day of the baby's life and with the traditional prayers and witnesses present so that the bris will still be considered kosher.

In terms of the bris celebration, I really wanted to do everything myself. I love entertaining and wanted everything to be just the way I like it. I didn't have a baby shower and wouldn't be throwing any other sort of welcoming party for our son, so I felt this was our one chance to really celebrate this baby's birth.

Eight days after a traumatic birth experience I wasn't able to be the head party planner and caterer I had envisioned, so instead I chose to focus on the things I really cared about: the ceremony and the cake. My husband and I really spent time writing a speech to share during the naming portion of the ceremony, and reading this aloud together that day is one of the moments I loved best about it. As for the cake—well, I spent months looking at Pinterest and chose a two-tiered round white cake with a light blue bowtie made of fondant wrapped around it and a cake topper with "Oh Boy" written in gold! Even with 80 guests, we had so much extra cake that we finished it at our son's birthday party a year later (you might want to save some space in your freezer).

Meg (who has twin 8-year-old boys and a 10-year-old son) comes from a Chinese background and is part of an interfaith couple. Her first experience with a Jewish bris took place when her first son was born. Many of the components of the ceremony were difficult and upsetting for her. She said her Chinese family thought some aspects of it were even quite funny from an outsider's perspective (a surgical procedure in the living room?), which she laughs about now. On the day of the event she was very emotional, and it was difficult to face such a big crowd and find something to wear so soon after giving birth. The mohel who performed the ceremony was also not helpful in comforting her or easing her experience on the day of the bris. She strongly recommends speaking with the mohel beforehand and being comfortable with them.

When it came time to having a bris for her twin sons, she decided to do the ceremony in a hospital without the party. For those who are undecided about what to do to, she recommends just keeping it intimate and small. Don't feel the need to invite dozens of friends and family members! You can still have a bris at home, or at the hospital, with just your closest family or friends.

Choosing a mohel

Before my baby was born I researched mohels in the area and spoke to them each briefly about their process. I asked them about how far in advance I would need to book them, how far they were willing to drive, etc. We ended up using one who is also a pediatric urologist, so that gave me some comfort. Many mohels today are not only trained in surgical circumcision but are also MDs themselves; so if that is a concern of yours you can probably find one in your area who has a medical background.

My biggest word of advice here is to find someone you feel comfortable with. Talk to them beforehand and ask them about what they do on the day of the ceremony and what you should expect. The purpose of this conversation is not just to get information but to get a good sense of who they are and whether they will be helpful leading you through the event.

We trusted our mohel 100% with the essential component of the day (the actual circumcision), but decided to ask our rabbi to join for the ceremony; we wanted to incorporate a longer and more spiritual side to the service and we had known him well for years. Don't forget to ask the mohel and rabbi for the fee they charge so you can have the money ready to pay them on the day of the event (it's like the wedding all over again!). There is a broad cost range depending on what part of the country you live in, but about $500 in a big city is pretty standard.

Rachel (whose kids are now 3, 6 and 9 years old) said that she really had very little concerns about her son's bris because she knew that she and her baby were in good hands with their mohel. He had performed the ceremony for her friends' babies and was well recommended in the area. She didn't need to think about the details of the ceremony because she trusted him to take care of all of it and this really helped her have one less thing to stress out about. So a good mohel can really be a blessing to the whole family!

What to ask a mohel

Here is a list of common things to ask your mohel about:

- ❑ How many circumcisions have you performed, and do you have references we can speak with?
- ❑ What religious denomination are you and how does this affect the ceremony?
- ❑ What pain relief do you recommend for the baby (before/during/after the circumcision)?
- ❑ After-care: how you recommend taking care of the penis after the circumcision? What are the signs of infection and what should we expect the area to look like afterwards?
- ❑ Use of shields and anesthesia for the baby: different mohels observe different practices when it comes to using a shield to protect the penis from the knife and using local anesthesia on the surgical site.
- ❑ What should the baby should wear for the ceremony?
- ❑ Who holds the baby when during the ceremony? Some mohels will hold the baby throughout the ceremony and afterwards while the parents share some words on the baby's name; some will give the baby to a relative to hold. Most parents don't worry or care about this detail, but if you're obsessed with details (like I am) you'll want to know!
- ❑ Who will speak and say the blessings? Can it be both parents, or just the father?
- ❑ What other honors are given out during the ceremony?
- ❑ When should the baby have his last feed before the bris?
- ❑ What ritual and practical items should the parents provide for the bris? (Usually you will need a tallis or two, a kiddush cup,

kosher wine, and candlesticks).

An important note: *"I heard that mohels sometimes orally suction the blood from the baby's penis; is this true?"*

I have heard this question before and it is a very important point to clarify: this practice is **not** commonly used in Jewish ceremonies. The practice is called *metzitzah b'peh*, and reports occasionally surface of it still being used in some ultra-Orthodox communities. Many mohels today have disavowed this practice. You might offend your mohel, but you can politely confirm that they do not practice this if you are concerned. Today to observe the mitzvah of the origination of this practice, mohels just check that blood flows out of the wound onto gauze.

When and where to have a bris

A bris should take place during daylight and most often occurs in the morning (usually fairly early, so people can get to work if it's during the weekday). However it is still kosher to have it later in the day, and many are also held after the workday. It is customary to have the bris at a time when more people can be there to witness it.

One nice thing about the bris is you have options when it comes to location! And options are a very nice thing when it comes to Jewish rituals, because sometimes there can be **a lot** of rules. It is customary to have a bris in a synagogue after morning prayers, but lots of people also have them at their homes, or even in a party space like a hotel or a restaurant.

We had a major debate in our family about where my son's bris would be held. I advocated the synagogue because the idea of arriving somewhere for the ceremony and going home afterwards had a lot of appeal — nothing to prep or cook or clean, no guests milling about my house, and no worries about escaping if I felt too tired or overwhelmed. I was also really freaked out about having a ton of people over to my home just days after I had a baby, knowing the place would be a mess, knowing I wouldn't have the time or energy to arrange things just as I wanted and knowing that I wouldn't have the privacy I needed figuring friends and family would want to come early and stay late.

Well as you probably have experienced by now, relationships and family involve a lot of compromise and in the end my husband cared so much about having it in our home that I gave in. And actually, it was lovely. Here's what really convinced me—I thought about my son. After going through this procedure, the idea of having to put the baby into a car and buckle a car seat so close to his sensitive area literally makes me shiver thinking about it.

I knew that the baby would be most comfortable if he was able to go straight into his own crib and not have to be moved again. Now a lot of mohels will tell you that after the procedure many babies go to sleep anyways and getting in a car seat is no trouble, but it's something to consider. As a concession my husband let me pick out an extravagant cake I had my eye on (have we talked enough about the cake yet!), and promised he would make sure all the food and table settings went where I wanted them to and that no one would be allowed into our bedroom if the door was closed. One other thing to consider though - remember that the table you use for the circumcision will likely remain in your home for many years - so if you don't mind having dinner where your baby was circumcised that's fine, but if it's going to bother you, consider using a different one! (It does have to be very sturdy and not the collapsible kind for obvious reasons).

If you've seen photos of a bris you've probably seen a table with a baby on it and a crowd of adults standing in the background. This is generally what they look like—standing room only. Unless you're going to have the ceremony at a synagogue you should not feel the need to provide seating for all your guests. People understand that this is not a sit-down formal event. The tradition goes back to ancient times when the whole village would join in the celebration and all were invited to partake in the joyous event. Also, it is traditional that during the actual ceremony everyone stands up to witness the holy event anyway.

It is customary to serve a meal to your guests after the bris. Because a bris is traditionally held in the morning, it's common to see foods like bagels and lox and different kugels served. There are no rules or specific foods that need to be there, and if your budget is tight consider keeping the menu to desserts and coffee, which is also fine.

Before the baby arrives you can think about what food you'd like to serve and get some prices and quotes together so that a lot of this legwork is done before the chaos of those first newborn days. I was able to determine a rough estimate of the number of people who would attend (I just did my best to guess at this) and then used that number to get price quotes from a few bagel places in our area. I didn't actually order anything but it made the planning process after my baby was here that much easier.

How to invite people to a bris

This is a tricky one! The date and time of a bris can't be determined until the baby is born, of course, because it has to take place exactly eight days after the birth. These eight days are calculated based on the Hebrew date of the baby's birth, meaning the day begins at sundown the night before. So if your baby is born on a Monday, his bris would be the following Monday. If he is born on a Monday evening after sunset (for example at 10 pm), the bris would take place on the following Tuesday. I've mentioned this earlier; but I do add it here again, because it is really confusing for many people!

Jewish parents really only have eight days maximum to plan and invite guests to the bris, and in reality it's actually fewer because it's hard to get much of anything done those first few days in the hospital aside from caring for the newborn and mom. Therefore mailing physical cards is very impractical. These days the most common way to announce the bris is by email or phone calls and often the message is combined with the birth announcement.

One other key custom to remember about informing guests about a bris is that a bris is a mitzvah, so it isn't something that you can technically *invite* someone to. Instead, people *announce* the time and location of the event to the family and friends whom they would like to attend. Along these same lines, it is customary not ask for RSVPs to the bris; but if you really do need firm numbers for catering, you can ask guests to RSVP to the meal after the bris for example to get around that.

Before the baby arrives is a good time to collect email addresses (as well as updated physical addresses for thank-you cards!) and gather together your list of who you'd like to share the details of the bris with. It can be a tough decision to determine how many people to invite (or technically **not** invite) to a bris. First, there are limits based on costs and location size. Renting a space and feeding guests can be cost-prohibitive for many families, and there are additional fees for the mohel to consider. Many people choose to only include their immediate family and closest friends because of these limitations. According to Jewish custom, no one should be excluded from a bris. If, in your heart, you want to open the event up to as many people as possible, then you can try to figure out a way to make that happen. However, the reality is that sometimes it just isn't possible and can be too overwhelming.

Rabbi Jaclyn Cohen of Temple Isaiah in West Los Angele remembers questioning whether or not to have a public circumcision for her new baby boy. She knew she wanted to celebrate with her congregation but wasn't sure whether or not to include everyone in a full bris ritual. When over 200 people attended she felt lifted up by the community, who were all there to share in the mitzvah and celebrate this new little life.

One really important reminder about your guests: a bris or baby naming can sometimes serve as the Jewish version of a baby shower. Gila Block who runs the Yesh Tikvah Jewish infertility organization reminded me that these events can be very emotional and triggering for a friend or family member who is struggling with infertility issues. Keep in mind that it's important to be kind and gentle and let these folks have the space they need if they choose not to attend your family's *simcha*. But it's really important to always include them and invite them, and then allow them to make the decision whether to attend.

What actually happens at a bris?

OK, here is real deal about what actually happens at a bris. From the shmoozing to the bagels and shmear, here is what you can expect to happen before during and after a bris.

Before

It's traditional for a bris to start on time, especially if it's in the morning before the workday starts; so people do their best to arrive on time. That being said, like any Jewish event, don't be surprised if things actually get started late. Generally the mohel will actually begin officiating the ceremony about 15-30 minutes after the time the bris is schedule just to give everyone enough time to arrive and get settled.

People generally dress in business casual attire to a bris and this is usually because it falls during the weekday before or after work hours; so people are just going to wear what they would normally wear to work. Slacks and a shirt or tie for men is fine, as is a suit; women generally wear a casual dress or slacks and a top. You can feel free to dress the same as your guests or to wear something a little nicer. Remember when you're thinking about your outfit that unless you are Kate Middleton you probably won't be able to walk around in heels so soon after giving birth and that your belly will still make you look about 4 or 5 months pregnant.

When people arrive they usually just chat standing up. If the bris is in someone's home, there isn't always seating for everyone—and there doesn't need to be. A bris is short and sweet and it's a mitzvah to stand during the actual ceremony.

The mom and baby are usually not around to welcome guests when they first arrive. The baby is being kept calm and quiet and away from large crowds and their germs since he is, of course, a newborn. The mohel will give you specific instructions about when to give the baby the last feed before the bris. It is common to have the father or grandparents around to greet guests. But if Dad prefers to be with Mom and baby, then delegate the task of greeting guests to someone else.

For a mom, it's nice to have this quiet time away from the commotion and nerves of the room. But if you are feeling social and excited to say hello to your friends and family who likely last saw you when you were still pregnant, it's perfectly OK to do so. Expect that you won't want to, though, as it is normal to be nervous, anxious and emotional on the day of the event.

The mohel will visit with the new parents before the ceremony and explain in detail what is about to happen and what to expect. The mohel should also go over detailed instructions with you for caring for the baby after the procedure; then he will go set up for the ceremony.

During

The first thing you may see is someone lighting candles—usually traditional Shabbat candles, but without saying a blessing. This is a traditional way of announcing to the community that a bris is being observed. During times when Jews were not allowed to freely practice their religion, this was a way of communicating to others in secret. Also, candlelight is often symbolic of the spark or miracle of God. The candle lighting is an honor of the ceremony and can be given to the mothers, grandmothers or great grandmothers of the baby.

The mother and father will bring the baby into the room and give him to the honorary figure chosen to actually carry the baby to the ceremony, called the *kvatter*. This is a special honor and it is usually given to the baby's uncle or grandfather. The mohel will welcome everyone in by sharing the words *baruch ha-bah*, which means welcome. Then the mohel will recite the Shema prayer.

Next the baby is placed on the "throne of Elijah," which is often a chair with a beautiful pillow or tallis placed on top of it. After that the baby is handed to the *sandek* who officially holds the baby during the circumcision. Generally the baby is placed either on a pillow or a device with a strap to hold him steady. The *sandek* will still spiritually hold the baby at this time but physically may just hold his foot, if anything at all. This is the highest honor of the bris and is usually given to the baby's grandfather.

Next the mohel recites:

> Here I am, ready to perform the commandment that the Creator has commanded us, to circumcise.

The next custom is for the baby's father to officially hand over the obligation (or mitzvah) of cicumcision to the mohel to perform on his behalf. You may find this exchange slightly humorous as the thought of the baby's actual father performing the circumcision is a little unsettling, but God commanded every father to circumcise their son, in the same way that Abraham circumsized his son Isaac (and himself at the age of 90!), So a father has to officially hadn over the mitzvah to the more qualified mohel (thank God for that!).

The mohel will then speak to the guests about the mitzvah of circumcision and may include some additional prayers or beautiful words about the family. Then he will prepare for the actual procedure which usually takes about 5-10 minutes.

After these prayers the actual circumcision will take place. During the circumcision the mohel uses an extremely sharp knife (designed to minimize pain) to remove the baby's foreskin. He then folds back the mucous membrane and exposes the glans of the penis.

During the actual circumcision it is not uncommon for the gathered crowd to chat to themselves and for the atmosphere to be quite lively. This may seem odd if you haven't attended a bris before, because you might expect total silence. But from my experience a mohel prefers not to have everyone silently staring at him as he works.

Once the mohel completes the circumcision the father (or parents) recites*: (*This can also be said as the mohel begins the circumcision depending on the mohel's partnership):

בָּרוּךְ אַתָּה אֲדֹנָי, אֱלֹהֵינוּ מֶלֶךְ הָעוֹלָם, אֲשֶׁר קִדְּשָׁנוּ בְּמִצְוֹתָיו וְצִוָּנוּ לְהַכְנִיסוֹ בִּבְרִיתוֹ שֶׁל אַבְרָהָם אָבִינוּ:

Baruch atah Adonai, Eloheinu Melech Ha'Olam, asher kideshanu be-mitzvotav vetzivanu lehochnisoh bivrito shel Avraham Avinu.

Blessed are You, Lord our God, King of the universe, Who has sanctified us with His commandments and commanded us to enter him into the Covenant of Abraham our father.

Then everyone responds:

כְּשֵׁם שֶׁהִכְנַסְתּוֹ לַבְּרִית, כָּךְ תִּזְכֶּה לְהַכְנִיסוֹ לַתּוֹרָה וְלַמִּצְוֹת וְלַחֻפָּה וּלְמַעֲשִׂים טוֹבִים

Ke-shem she-nich-nas la-brit kein yi-ka-neis-o le-to-rah le-choo-pah oo-le-ma-a-sim to-vim.

Just as he has entered into the Covenant, so may he enter into Torah, into marriage, and into good deeds.

Afterwards

After the actual circumcision is performed, the baby is wrapped in a clean diaper and the mohel will hand the baby over to the *standing sandek* at this time, which is another very special honor. The mohel (or rabbi) will then say two more prayers; then, lifting the kiddush cup of wine, will announce the baby's name for the first time. Traditionally this is when everyone learns the baby's name and hears it for the first time. Many parents share the English name when the baby is first born and save the reveal of the Hebrew name for the bris.

Next the parents are invited to share a prepared speech about the child's name. This is usually just a few paragraphs long and tells the story of the people the baby was named for. Don't be surprised if the baby starts to cry around this time. The baby is usually given a few drops of wine or the mohel will wrap gauze around his finger and dip it in wine and let the baby suck on it. Keep in mind that your baby will want to nurse and sleep after all this so do try to keep your prepared speech on the shorter side!

Finally, it's time to eat—which is actually a critical part of observing the mitzvah of *brit milah*!

When the ceremony is finished and guests head to the food, Mom—and sometimes Dad—head off to feed and calm the baby. Generally after nursing and some pain relief, the baby will fall asleep and won't remember a thing. For the new parents it should be a day they remember as full of joy.

What will the baby be like after the bris?

It can take a few minutes for the baby to get upset. Many people are surprised that there often isn't much crying during the circumcision itself. Depending on the pain relief (usually Tylenol) and numbing agent the baby is often sore and tired a little after the experience. I have found that 15 or so minutes after the circumcision the baby will really start to get upset. At this point the official bris components should be over and guests should be making their way to the *seuda* meal. Mom and baby usually leave right away to go to a quiet place to give the mom a chance to calm, comfort and feed the baby.

It's best to play loud white noise for them (in a pinch type in 'white noise for babies' on YouTube and play one of the videos!), which mimics sounds in the womb, and swaddle them snuggly so that their legs are not kicking around which could aggravate the situation. Next try rocking them in a rocking chair or bouncing on an exercise ball to help them calm down. When they are calm enough nurse or feed them and they should fall asleep quite easily and sleep for a nice long while. Make sure to talk to the mohel if you are concerned or need help calming them. Expect them to take a bit longer to calm down than they usually would and that they may not latch right away if they're very upset. Many babies will also need to be burped as they'll swallow a lot of air during the ceremony and afterwards.

Ritual objects you'll need for a bris

Your mohel should provide you with detailed instructions about what to prepare or bring with you to the ceremony. Here is a quick list to give you an overview of what to expect:

❏ Chair for Elijah
❏ Candles (often the families use their Shabbat candlesticks)
❏ Kiddush cup
❏ Tallis

Your mohel should also provide a list of other things necessary on the day of the bris, for example Tylenol, extra diapers, and instructions on what he would like the baby to wear.

As mentioned in the previous section, there are also a few honors to give out at the bris; so take some time to think about who those special family and friends are who you would like to be involved:

Kvatter: this honor is usually given to a married couple without children of their own. They bring the baby into the room.

The baby is also placed on Elijah's chair, taken off the chair, and held for blessings afterwards. You can assign people for each of these honors as well or just have the *kvatter* perform them.

Sandek: this is the highest honor and it is traditionally given to the baby's grandfather. The sandek holds the baby during the circumcision.

Standing Sandek: After the ceremony, this person will hold the baby.

Prayers/Readings: If you would like to honor additional family members, you can assign them prayers or readings.

Can you take photos at a bris?

Yes! Lots! The mohel will warn you about moments in the ceremony where photos are not allowed—including when the baby is on Elijah's chair, and during the actual circumcision. So just make sure to ask the mohel beforehand and he will usually know to instruct the guests in attendance the same thing. If you're wondering about some posed family photos, you may want to make some time for these before your other guests arrive. The closer to bris time it is, the more stress and emotion you will likely be feeling. After the bris, the baby will need to feed and rest.

Special considerations for premature infants and honoring a difficult conception and pregnancy journey

For a baby who is born prematurely, figuring out when and how to have a bris can be a complicated manner. Jessica Copeland, whose son is now one year old, shared her experience with me. Her son was born at 29 weeks and one day gestational age. She had been diagnosed with preeclampsia and her baby was Intrauterine Growth Restricted, meaning he was very small. When he was born via C-section, Zach weighed just 1lb. 7.8 oz and measured 13.11 inches long.

Here is the story of his naming and bris as told by Jessica:

> The most common question we were asked in the hospital in the antipartum, postpartum and NICU stages was, "What is his name?" Our answer was, "The baby

has no name." While all of the babies in the NICU had cute signs taped to their isolettes with their names written in fun letters and their birthdate and weight decorated with stickers and cute scrapbook paper, "Falafel" (the nickname my husband and I gave him) had a blank sign with his birthdate and weight and length. The paper was cute, but both nurses and doctors alike looked super confused and often turned the laminated sheet over and searched around the small NICU bed space searching for the name of our child. For 9 days he had no name; for 9 days we were asked what his name was and when he would have one; for 9 days we struggled to come up with a name. Were we supposed to name him? Were we allowed to name him? Would we call him Falafel until he was circumcised at his bris?

According to Jewish tradition a baby boy is circumcised in a religious ceremony on their 8th day of life. At that time the child is given their name and presented to the community. A 1 lb 7.8 oz baby cannot be circumcised. The policy of the NICU is that they do the circumcision right before the baby is discharged from the hospital. So we had to wait for him to be circumcised. Were we going to have to call our child Falafel for the foreseeable future? Would he be scared for life? To the internet we went!

There was such a lack of information about what to do in this situation. How many people have micro preemies? How many of those micro preemies are boys? How many of those boys' parents feel that it is crucial for them to be circumcised and named according to Jewish law and customs?

We ended up reaching out to the rabbi at the shul in Columbus, where we lived. He had to do some research and talk to fellow rabbis about the issue. He came back to us with the following: If the baby is expected to live and leave the hospital it can be given a name. If there is any doubt whether the child will survive, you must wait until you are sure in order to give them a name.

We sheepishly approached one of the residents and explained the situation and basically straight out had to ask if our child was going to survive and be released from the hospital at some point in the future. She was definitely taken aback but emphatically stated with certainty that our child would be discharged at some point in the future! This meant that we could give Falafel a name less reminiscent of a delicious fried food item.

But how do you give a Jewish baby boy his name if you are not having a bris? The answer is that the father (in the Orthodox tradition father only—I'm sure it would likely be both the mother and father in other traditions) is given an Aliyah (called up to the Torah) during the morning service. After saying the prayers and listening to the Torah reading, the rabbi says a prayer that is part of what is said at a bris and announces the name of the child.

So we called our family and told them that we were going to be naming our child during the morning minyan on Thursday June 8th. We answered many questions: No, he wasn't going to be there. No, he wasn't going to get circumcised. No, the rabbi didn't have to go to the hospital and bless the baby. It was a short service. A few of our family members came and our son was named. We didn't tell our family beforehand what the name was, so they were all surprised when the rabbi announced our son as Zachary Samson Copeland—*Zachariah Shimshon*. After the service, we ate bagels at our house and then headed to the hospital to officially tell them our son's legal name.

The actual circumcision took place once Zach came

home from the hospital. We had the unique opportunity to select the date for his bris—which was nice, since most of our family lived out of town. We contacted the mohel in Columbus and he was a bit wary of our request to book him for three weeks in advance, and he was very confused when we told him that our son was 3 months old but only about 6 pounds. Thankfully, he was more than happy to perform the circumcision. So on September 17, 2017, 109 days after Zach was born, our family came together and he was circumcised.

If you have a preemie or a micro-preemie baby and have questions about what to do, I hope Jessica's story gives you hope and comfort. There are resources and answers out there and hopefully a name and a Jewish identity can be one of those milestones in those early scary days that your baby really is here and really is yours.

Gila Block, Executive Director and cofounder of the Yesh Tikva organization which supports Jewish families through infertility, told me that when her daughter was born she wanted to do something beyond the traditional ceremony. She wanted to celebrate the enormous feeling of gratitude and celebration she felt at finally having a baby after a long journey through infertility.

She and her family decided to have a *Simchat Hodaya*, which translates to the Joy of Thanksgiving. In Judaism this term is used to describe a party to celebrate when something truly wonderful and miraculous happens to you, to give thanks for something like being in remission from cancer or surviving a car accident. It often celebrates the good that can come from something bad. It also honors those in the room who have been on the journey as well; these events often affect the extended family and community.

For Gila, everyone in the room was invited to share their thoughts and feelings at reaching this milestone and it elevated the day and made it that much more special to hear their words. She described it as a "special way to take a step back from the business of raising a newborn and remember what it took get there: a four-year journey and four IVF cycles." For her it was a time "to memorialize and to be thankful."

Simchat Bat, celebrating a girl!

Don't worry, boys don't get to have all the fun! There are some beautiful options for celebrating a baby girl, and there's a lot more flexibility in terms of location and timing for the event. There are even different names for the celebration: *Simchat bat* means "Rejoicing in a Daughter" and is the most popular one; but people also use *brit bat,* or "daughter's covenant," to keep the similarity to a boy's *brit milah.* Sephardic Jews use the term *zeved bat* or "gift of a daughter" and usually hold the ceremony in the first month after the daughter's birth.

For timing, if you plan to involve a rabbi you should speak with them about when they traditionally have naming ceremonies for girls. The most common times are one month after the child is born (30 days after birth was in ancient times when a baby was considered to be viable and completely have a life of their own) or three months after they are born (the length of time the Torah recommends to wait before the mother would bring sacrifices to the Temple after the birth of a girl). The beginning of a new Hebrew month, called *Rosh Chodesh*, is also a symbolic time associated with women; so often the first of the new Hebrew month is the date chosen for the celebration.

For location the customs are similar to a bris: it is traditionally held in the synagogue or family home. What's nice about the synagogue is the service already provides a minyan, and a religious event for people to participate in which the naming can be incorporated into. If you choose to have the ceremony in your home it may take some additional consideration over which prayers and other readings to include in the ceremony. If the celebration takes place during a summer month there are also many families who choose to host the celebration outdoors and even incorporate music and dancing into it. Like a boy's bris, you can include traditional ritual objects like a Kiddush cup to say the blessing over the wine (traditional at most joyous celebrations) and a tallit (prayer shawl) to wrap the baby.

Because a naming ceremony for a girl doesn't have the same *halachic* traditions stipulating exactly what must take place like a bris does, you can embrace your creativity in planning the event. You have more time and flexibility to plan it and you can work with your rabbi to create a ceremony that is meaningful to you. This is especially true if you're hosting the event in your home and not during morning services at synagogue.

The core element of sharing the baby's English and Hebrew name is the heart of the celebration, so it's traditional to share the meaning behind the name and the positive characteristics of the person she is named for. After the naming ceremony it's traditional to serve guests a meal just like you would at a bris.

Some advice from real moms on the bris

Here are some snippets of advice from real moms about having a bris:

Debbie, whose children are 35 and 31 years old, told me that "It's always lovely to try to incorporate family traditions and/or religious items (kiddush cup, tallit, kippot, challah cover, etc.) into your child's bris or baby naming. My parents were Holocaust survivors and my dad was able to bring with him, out of Germany, his handmade bris gown. That bris gown has now lovingly been worn by 3 grandsons and five great-grandsons. As with any other beautiful event, try to make it about the meaning of the event and not get so wrapped up in the party itself."

Tiffany (Instagram handle *@raisingbumbles*) whose children are 6 and 2 said, "Ours was very untraditional. We waited until after the birth of my son to have the naming ceremony for both our daughter and son at the same time. She was four at the time. My son was circumcised in the hospital, so our bris was very relaxed. Our rabbi was so great! We met with her while I was pregnant with my son and we explained that my son had been diagnosed with a medical condition while in utero and it was very important for us to have a bris. She was the one who suggested we include my daughter as well. She was so helpful in helping us plan it and since I had never been to one (I just never had the chance to attend one growing up), she helped explain what was involved to both me and my husband (who is not Jewish) and made the experience very easy. She gave us options for prayers and readings to choose from. And she checked in with me a lot to see if I had any questions or concerns."

Shawna, whose son is now almost 4, said her best advice is, "Get a mohel who makes you feel comfortable. I was extremely apprehensive about the bris but our mohel was amazing and really put me at ease. Also, accept help when people offer!!"

What about baby #2, #3 etc.

In terms of celebrations, each life is a unique gift! If you are feeling like you don't want to host another major event, it is fine to invite fewer guests, have the celebration just be part of a morning service at the synagogue, or specify "no gifts" on the invitation.

Another thing to consider is how to include your older children in the event. You may have a toddler or preschooler who is just getting used to the idea of having a newborn around, so talk to them beforehand about what is going to happen. Let them know there will be a lot of people and it is like a party for their new sibling. You can either designate someone like an aunt or uncle to be their special buddy during the ceremony or have them join you at the front with the mohel or rabbi. You may also want to consider having a present ready for them for after the party as they will likely see their new sibling being given lots of new things.

Some mohels and rabbis will be encouraging of including older children in the ceremony itself. If children are old enough they can read a short prayer, or they can help hold the baby before the ceremony. There are also some very creative ideas like having older children say a blessing for the baby, present them with a homemade card, or sprinkle flower petals on them.

So you don't want to have a bris or maybe even a circumcision. What's the alternative?

While having a traditional bris is still very much the norm even for less observant Jewish families, there are parents who are opposed to the idea of the bris and even the circumcision itself. While this choice may seem taboo for many Jewish families and it is rare that a rabbi would officiate at a religious ceremonial alternative, there are some families who assert that this ancient custom violates the identity and freedom of the baby.

Those families may choose to do a *brit shalom* instead of a bris for a boy, which resembles the naming ceremony for a girl. A *brit shalom* (a Covenant of Peace) may include rituals like washing the baby's feet in water. This is an ancient Biblical practice described in the story of Abraham, used to welcome guests. After Abraham's guests arrived he welcomed them into his home by washing their feet. His wife Sarah, who had thus far been unable to have children, was finally able to conceive after this visit.

Some families choose to leave the foreskin intact and observe a *hatefet dam brit* instead (more on that below). If you are considering this you do need to take into account that most Jewish rabbis and congregations do not consider this an equal replacement for a Bris if the foreskin is left intact and consider it instead a "waste of blood."

You may hear the term "kinder cut," which refers to a partial circumcision in which only the very tip of the foreskin—the part extending past the acorn shaped head of the penis—is removed. This is a medically discouraged practice; the skin can heal in a way that adheres to the penis, which is dangerous and may require surgery to repair. Again, this type of circumcision is not considered "kosher" or having fulfilled the mitzvah by most branches of Judaism.

If you are feeling unsure about circumcising your son at all, you are not alone. Attitudes in America are shifting. In 2012 the American Academy of Pediatrics stated that while the benefits outweigh the risks, they no longer recommend "universal newborn circumcision." The scientific community as a whole is not in total agreement, either; although some studies have shown that circumcision can help prevent penile cancer, UTIs and STDs like HIV.

If you are sure that you do not want to circumcise but are concerned about what life will be like for an uncircumcised Jewish boy growing up, you may want to visit BeyondtheBris.com, a small online community for these families.

So you didn't have a bris on the 8th day. Is it too late?

If a baby was circumcised in a hospital, or before becoming Jewish (so they had a non-religious circumcision), or they are converting to Judaism after birth and are not circumcised at all, a *hatefet dam brit* ceremony can take place instead. This ceremony which means "shedding of blood" is a ritualistic circumcision in which a mohel draws just a drop of blood from the penis so that the commandment can be officially observed. The Reform movement does not require the physical act to be performed on boys or men who are converting to Judaism.

12.

A Spiritual Birth Plan

The day you were born
is the day God decided that the world could not exist without you.
—Rabbi Nachman of Breslov

Special words in the Hebrew language have meaning woven into their letters. The word for "womb" in Hebrew is *be-rechem*. The root of the word *rechem* means mercy and compassion. Intrinsically, a mother has a deep and ancient connection to her baby, and during birth the concepts of mercy and compassion really come to fruition. As a mother who personally suffered a traumatic birth experience when my son as born two years ago, I know firsthand how a woman in labor is at the mercy and control of others around her. My attention was so solely focused on bringing my baby into this world that I had little compassion for myself, or for my own emotional experience during the birth. It is only through unpacking the events in my mind months later that I realized how unfair this was.

One of the most surprising aspects of Jewish tradition is its absenteeism during childbirth. Although Judaism is rich in prayer and *minhag* (custom) during almost every other significant life cycle event, there is no religious ritual for women during the birth experience. Maybe it's because our sages were male, and because women aren't bound by the same time-bound *mitzvot* as men. As a result we are left with what can be a life-altering experience devoid of spiritual support.

My intention in this chapter is reclaim a sense on control and agency during the birth process—at least in spiritual terms!

There have been many of studies of faith, meditation and hypnosis during childbirth and how creating a calm and spiritual environment encourages the mother and helps to progress labor. If you are interested in learning more about the effect of these ancient practices on labor, I really recommend researching these techniques.

There's a very helpful book called *Hypnobirthing: The Mongan Method*, by Marie Mongan, which goes into a lot of research on the power of the mind to not only calm the mother but also to create a more positive birthing experience. Her book talks about alleviating fear and training the mind to activate certain areas of the body to help the baby emerge. While this book is not about Judaism, it does speak to spirituality and ancient tradition and reinforces the idea that as a woman, you **already** know how to birth and you are ready, you are capable, and you do not need to be afraid of the experience.

In Biblical times, women gave birth assisted by only a midwife. During the births of ancient times, much emphasis was placed on connecting to the spiritual aspects of Mother Nature and finding each new mother's place in this manifestation of life.

The Chassidic and Kabbalistic communities consider labor to be a time of judgement; in order to bring about the best outcome they use song, dance, and prayer. When wives go into labor, their husbands and communities will spend the time rejoicing in prayer and raising their voices in song—thanking God and saying blessings for the woman in labor.

They also believe that crying out to God during labor—especially during the time of pushing the baby out—awakens God's mercy and is a special sound and prayer that God can hear. In this way the baby is born hearing his mother's special prayer to God. The act of labor is a way of surrendering to God or to the larger powers of fate in the universe with an acceptance that we cannot control everything in our lives.

The spirituality of birth in Judaism

Some Jewish women believe that we are meant to suffer in childbirth, that this is our punishment as descendants of Eve. In her essay "Sacred Screaming," Lori Hope Lefkovitz talks about how childbirth in Judaism is full of contradictions. On one hand, there's this sense of pain, suffering, and punishment; but on the other, we're fulfilling God's most emphasized commandment in the Torah—to be fruitful and multiply. In Eve's story, after the serpent entices her to eat the forbidden fruit, God says to her, "I will make most severe Your pangs in childbearing; In pain shall you bear children." (Genesis 3:16). If only every diet plan came with that kind of motivation—not that it worked for Eve!

When Jewish law was codified hundreds of years ago, the rabbis were focused on the laws of purity surrounding childbirth, and not the spirituality or experience of the women giving birth. Throughout their writings you find contradictions between the notions of fulfilling a great mitzvah but also sharing Eve's punishment. As a result, many Jewish women today find nothing useful in these ancient writings for their own birth experiences.

When I packed my hospital bag I put in a siddur and a *B'kol Echad* (a Jewish song book), thinking that I might have time to pray during labor and delivery. I paused as I placed it neatly into my little curated carry-on, because I wasn't sure which prayers I should actually remember to say. As it turns out, I never did open either one. I think part of the reason for that is I had no idea which prayers to turn to. As I am pregnant again now, I want to create a ritual to comfort and care for myself during what I know will be one of the most significant days of my life.

I spoke to Rabbi Sara Brandes, Executive Director at Or Ha-Lev: Center for Jewish Spirituality and Meditation, and part of the Shechinah Counsel of rabbinic and Jewish educational advisors for At the Well, and I asked her if she felt there was a Jewish spiritual component to birth. She responded that there "absolutely should be!" She told me about her friend who sang through her delivery!

Rabbi Sara told me that Judaism has a lot to say about "humility, gratitude, softening, protection and transition—all essential elements of the birth process." There are also many symbolic references to birth woven throughout Judaism, which both acknowledges and honors the process. The story of the Jewish people needing to leave Egypt to cross narrow watery straits and arrive at the promised land is a key one. The mikvah itself also represents the womb, and every time we enter it we are, in a sense, reborn again. So if you look at ancient Jewish texts through the lens of a modern woman, there are components of spirituality and connections to pregnancy all around us.

I spoke to Author and Rabbi Nina Beth Cardin about a book she wrote called *Out of the Depths I Call to You: A Book of Prayers for the Married Jewish Woman*, in which she translates and explains prayers and psalms from an 18th-century Italian prayer book that was specifically for women. This illuminating resource shows that, throughout our history, there have been times when Judaism was full of spiritual support for the birth experience.

Sacred birth—midwives in Judaism

Midwives have an ancient and mystical reputation in Judaism; we hear stories of them throughout the Bible. In the Torah portion *Shemot* we meet two of the most well-known and pioneering female Biblical figures: Shifra and Puah. In Egypt, the story goes that Pharaoh was afraid of the Jewish people whom he had enslaved because their numbers continued to multiply. He commanded the two midwives to kill all Jewish baby boys that were born. But despite the danger, they feared God more than the Pharaoh and disobeyed his commands.

These women are not only powerful role models in Judaism; they exemplify some of the first examples of females leading a resistance against a tyrannical regime. In the Torah they are rewarded for their righteous actions directly by God.

Much of the *midrashim* (stories and commentary) written by rabbis on these two women also delves into the sacred knowledge that midwives have of how to safely bring mother and baby through the birthing process. Even their names are intertwined with some of these caring and sacred acts. For example, the word *shiprah* is connected to the Hebrew word *meshaperet*, which means *to beautify or cleanse*; one of the midwives' great honors was to wash the newborn babies after they were born. The word *puah* is also interpreted as *to cry*, because the midwives held a unique knowledge of not only how to bring a healthy baby into the world (a crying baby meant it was alive and strong) but also how to comfort them. Another interpretation is that the word *sheparu*, which is synonymous with *fruitful*, comes from their names because they allowed the Israelites to be fruitful and multiply.

Shifra and Puah are also said to have spoken special prayers to God, asking for God's assistance in bringing each baby into the world safely and in good health. In this way they were active partners with God and the mother in the very act of creation. Without the help of the midwives, Yocheved would not have been able to birth Moses; so in many ways, the fate of the Jewish people was literally in their hands that day. Their actions were the very start of delivering the Jewish people from exile and into the promised land.

Today there are Jewish doulas who are engaged in these very same acts of protecting mothers and babies during birth.

Jewish birth workers today

Many women consider hiring a professional doula, or birth worker, to support them during their labor and delivery. A doula can offer support throughout a pregnancy as well as provide postpartum care, but they are most often brought in during the labor experience. For women who want a natural or unmedicated delivery, whether that's in a hospital, birth center, or their home, a doula can help in a way that nurses and doctors can't. For example, a doula can come to a woman's home and coach them through their contractions throughout labor. What this coaching entails can vary depending on the style and training of your doula, but generally they work with the mother to find comfortable positions, work through pain management strategies, and help her achieve the birth plan she desires.

I spoke to Na'amah Wendy Kenin, the founding doula of Imeinu Doulas and Jewish Birth Collective, who coordinates a professional network of Jewish birth workers around the world. She explained that "Doulas are resources who can give mothers holistic support." Imeinu has now expanded beyond just doulas and midwives to include acupuncture, nutrition counseling, and postpartum counseling to create an entire support team for pregnant women.

To provide a Jewish experience as a doula, Na'amah told me how she pulls from various sources like prayer and the Torah to create a "Jewish spiritual orientation around childbirth and postpartum support." These practices can range from performing a ritual hand-washing ceremony for the mom after the childbirth to specific prayers for the first time the baby breastfeeds. A Jewish doula can also be present for a mother at the mikvah during the last month of her pregnancy. Doulas can even facilitate a ceremony for her and her friends or a group of women to heighten the spiritual experience of the mikvah. Na'amah also talked to me about the specific training she shares when working with women who have suffered pregnancy loss, encouraging them to go through a "personal rebirth"—especially surrounding returning to the mikvah and associating with life once again.

Rabbi and doula Denise Handlarski of the SecularSyngagogue. com is part of Imeinu Doulas. She told me that she saw the necessity of combining birth work with Judaism through her own labor and delivery experiences—which didn't go as she had planned. As a rabbi, Jewish tradition played such an important role in her life; but her birth experience lacked a Jewish connection, which made her feel like this important part of who she was wasn't there in the way she needed it to be.

Today she works to enable moms to have a "successful birth," which for her means not just "a healthy baby and a healthy person who gave birth," but also that the person who gave birth "feels that they were seen, and got to maintain a sense of control." She tries to make birth not just a medical experience but something that taps into who the woman is as a whole and honors that. Part of the way she enables that is to help her clients learn and prepare for birth. Panic and fear exacerbate pain; the more women know about what is going to happen, the less fear they will have.

Na'mah and the doulas she works with are also focused on postpartum care. She explained that, particularly in the U.S., women are "often left without support" after giving birth. Part of what makes working with her different from a "normal" labor and delivery experience is that after birth she helps moms create a plan for how they are going to eat, stay hydrated, stay healthy and have support around the house.

If you are interested in finding a doula who is part of the Imeinu network, you can visit their website (imeinu.wordpress.com/). They also specialize in working with unique Jewish families—LGBT families and families who identify as gender queer or gender fluid and are focused on social justice in the birth community.

How to create a spiritual birth plan

There are few things women get to have total control of in the birthing process. Even the most detailed birth plan can be tossed aside if the baby's heart rate slows or the baby decides to flip positions. I didn't have much of a birth plan aside from two things. First, I wanted to have skin to skin contact as soon as the baby was born; and second, I wanted to delay cord clamping. These were both things I had researched heavily and felt were best for the health and wellbeing of me and my child. Although I was unfortunate in a lot of the birth experience with my son (well, really the healing afterwards) I did get to have these two elements. I made them very clear to my husband, nurses, and doctors, and made sure ahead of time that the hospital, doctors, and nursing staff supported these practices. So, although birth plans sometimes get a bad rap for being unrealistic, I actually found that making a plan and clarifying for yourself and your support team what you want can help push things in that direction.

I wasn't prepared with a spiritual birth plan that time, but this time will be different. My spiritual birth plan with my second baby is to keep it simple. In this chapter I'm going to help you create yours.

I know from experience that I may not have long stretches of time to read or recite something, so when active labor really begins and I head to the hospital I will simply say the *shema* prayer—the same prayer I sing to my son each night before he falls asleep. Each night I use that time to ask God to watch over him during the night, and I'll use the prayer to ask God to watch over me during the unknowns of my time in the hospital bringing my baby into this world.

Then, when—God-willing—the baby is here, I will say the *she-hecheyanu*—the same prayer I recited when I found out I was pregnant and what I will say when I immerse in the mikvah at my ninth month. I'll say it to thank God for sustaining me through a long nine months of pregnancy, keeping me alive during the dangers of birth and enabling me to reach such a blessed day as to see my baby come into this world. Here are the words of the Shehecheyanu prayer as translated by Chabad:

בָּרוּךְ אַתָּה אַדֹנָי אֱלֹהֵינוּ מֶלֶךְ הָעוֹלָם, שֶׁהֶחֱיָנוּ וְקִיְּמָנוּ וְהִגִּיעָנוּ לַזְּמָן הַזֶּה

Baruch atah, Adonai Eloheinu, Melech haolam,
shehecheyanu, v'kiy'manu, v'higiyanu laz'man hazeh.

Blessed are You, Lord our God, King of the Universe, who has granted us life, sustained us and enabled us to reach this occasion.

I spoke to Rabbi Stuart Weinblatt of Temple B'nai Tzedek in Maryland, who shared with me that he and his wife said the *she-*

hecheyanu prayer when each of his children were born. He told me that he chose to do this because he wanted the first words that they heard to be words of blessing. He considers the prayer to be beautiful and wanted to thank God for bringing him and his family to that day and moment in time.

I was curious to know more about why birth related prayers and rituals aren't more defined in Jewish tradition, and author Anita Diamant had a very profound answer for me. She told me that the experience of giving birth is "sacred in itself". She said that "if you're present for that moment (birth), then you're present for the most sacred moment in life". Birth itself is so miraculous, and so spiritual that it is in a way beyond ritual and prayer. And because this moment is so unequal in its holiness, our ability to add words of prayer to it are unnecessary. In moments like these, Anita explained, "language fails" because it just can't compete with what's going on, birth is beyond words.

On your way to the hospital or as labor begins

There are many "good luck" Jewish traditions you can incorporate into your spiritual birth plan if they appeal to you. You can wear or hold a hamsa charm—an ancient symbol of a hand meant to keep the *evil eye* away. You can also wear a red string (discussed in detail in Chapter 6) which also is said to be a connection to God and a protection from evil spirits.

You can also use this time to sing Jewish prayers, to dance to Jewish music like Israeli folk dancing, and to just use the sights and sounds of Judaism to put you in the right state of mind for the momentous event of labor and delivery. It's best to plan ahead and tap into what you know resonates with you so that you can have these items on hand.

Support in the room

Part of your spiritual birth plan should include the physical elements that can provide you with emotional support during labor and delivery. This can include things like adjusting the lighting in the room (you can sometimes request to soften or turn down the lights while the doctors aren't in the room), or having music playing. If Jewish music or prayers are meaningful to you, I encourage you to make a playlist and include them to help invite a sense of uplifting spiritual feeling in the room. Rabbi Handlarski suggested including Jewish art in your room to help evoke positive feelings.

Rabbi Handlarski also shared with me that one of the ways she supports her clients is by helping them create a refrain or affirmation to repeat through the labor process. For example: *Kol haolam kuloh, gesher tzar m'od. V'haikar lo l'facheid k'lal.* This beginning of this famous Jewish quote means, *the whole world is a narrow bridge.* The second line of the quote says *the most important thing is not to be afraid.* The connection between these words and the physical birth process is meaningful, and the message of strength and bravery can be empowering and helpful for women.

The one thing you can definitely control is who is in the room with you. As we discuss in Chapter 8, Jewish moms and mothers-in-law have a semi-deserved reputation for being especially involved in their children's (and grandchildren's!) lives, and you may get a request, plea or outright demand for them to be present in the hospital room. If you believe these loving family members will support you, help you, calm you and encourage you, then it can be a true blessing to have them there. If, however, you don't want them to be there, that is your right to decide.

When the baby arrives—blessing the child

When the baby arrives, the most common thing to say is "*Mazal Tov!*" and in Orthodox circles you'll hear the "*hatov ve'hametiv*" prayers for a boy, which means *God does good.* When Eve gave birth she said "I have been given a child, with the help of God."

Medical research now confirms the benefits of skin-to-skin contact. That means that when the baby first arrives it's best for them to be placed on the mother's bare chest so her body warmth and soothing touch can calm and comfort them in their first few minutes in the world. This can be a very spiritual experience and if it's important to you, you should let the doctors and nurses know that you would like to have this special bonding time be as uninterrupted as possible. Know that there may be some stitches and placenta birthing to be done, but in the chaos there are also moments of beautiful calm of just mama and baby, and it's beneficial for both to be physically connected during this time. This is a lovely moment to offer a blessing to your child and share with them whether silently or aloud how loved they are.

In Jewish tradition a baby is born pure and without sin. Unlike in many Christian traditions, Jews believe there is no need to baptize them or say any prayers in the hopes of removing sin from them. There is even an old Jewish story that babies spend the time in the womb learning the whole Torah, then before they are born an angel wipes the knowledge away and this is what causes the little groove in our upper lip—the philtrum. It is where an angel touched each of us.

There are some verses that are traditionally said at the time of birth, including Psalm 126, which includes the words, "Those who sow in tears will reap in joy" and Psalm 118, which speaks about coming close to death but trusting in God to answer our prayers. Yet there are no specific prayers to say when you go into labor or even when the baby is born. However, Judaism is additive and inclusive and if creating a spiritual birth plan is something you feel would add positively to your experience then it is absolutely something you should create and bring with you to the hospital.

Other Jewish traditions include singing the Shir Hamaalot prayer for a new mother or hanging it in her room at the hospital. This prayer is believed to offer protection for her and her baby, exposing the child to holy words and prayer as part of the first thing he experiences in the world.

The traditional prayer for a child is the one recited on Shabbat as the candles are lit each Friday night. The prayer asks for boys to be like Ephrayim and Menasheh and girls to grow to be like Sarah, Rebecca, Rachel and Leah. These prayers can be another beautiful option to share with your baby when they arrive into the world, the translations below are taken from Ritualwell.

For children

יְבָרֶכְךָ אֲדֹנָי וְיִשְׁמְרֶךָ.
יָאֵר אֲדֹנָי פָּנָיו אֵלֶיךָ וִיחֻנֶּךָּ.
יִשָּׂא אֲדֹנָי פָּנָיו אֵלֶיךָ וְיָשֵׂם לְךָ שָׁלוֹם.

Ye'varech'echa Adonoy ve'yish'merecha.
Ya'ir Adonoy panav eilecha viy-chuneka.
Yisa Adonoy panav eilecha, ve'yasim lecha shalom.

May God bless you and watch over you.
May God shine His face toward you and show you favor.
May God be favorably disposed toward you and grant you peace.

For a boy

יְשִׂמְךָ אֱלֹהִים כְּאֶפְרַיִם וְכִמְנַשֶּׁה

Ye'simcha Elohim ke-Ephraim ve'chi-Menashe.

May God make you like Ephraim and Menashe.

For a girl

יְשִׂימֵךְ אֱלֹהִים כְּשָׂרָה, רִבְקָה, רָחֵל וְלֵאָה.

Ye'simech Elohim ke-Sarah, Rivka, Ra-chel ve-Lay'ah.

May God make you like Sarah, Rebecca, Rachel and Leah.

We ask God for our children to be like Ephraim and Menashe because, in the Torah, just before Jacob dies he blesses them and foretells how they will be a blessing to all of Israel (Genesis 48:20). These two boys were the sons of Joseph, but were given this special blessing by Joseph's own father, Jacob. Unlike previous stories of rival brothers in the Bible, these two were the first to live together in harmony. We ask for God to bless our girls to be like the matriarchs of the Bible, who each had their own heroic journeys and are exemplary figures of holiness and blessing.

These same prayers are used when people embark on a long or difficult journey, so it's appropriate if we think of all of life as a journey and ask God to bless this child on their very first day of it.

Coming home from the hospital and a blessing for Mom

After the baby has arrived safely and the mom is healthy, it's traditional for her partner (or both parents together) to recite the *Birkat Hagomel*, which is a prayer traditionally recited to thank God when we have survived a perilous journey. It is common to recite this prayer at synagogue in the presence of a minyan after the Torah is read. Here are the words of the Birkat Hagomel prayer for the new mother to recite, as translated by Ritualwell:

בָּרוּךְ אַתָּה אֲדֹנָי אֱלֹהֵינוּ מֶלֶךְ הָעוֹלָם
הַגוֹמֵל לְחַיָּבִים טוֹבוֹת שֶׁגְּמָלַנִי כָּל טוֹב

Barukh Atah Adonay Eloheynu Melekh Ha'olam,
hagomel li-khayavim tovot shegamalni kol tov.

Blessed are You, oh Lord, our God, King of the universe who bestows goodness upon the accountable, who has bestowed every goodness upon me.

When recited in the synagogue, the congregation responds:

מִי שֶׁגְמָלְךָ כֹּל טוֹב הוּא יִגְמָלְךָ כֹּל טוֹב סֶלָה

Amen. Mi shegamalech tov, Hu yig'malech kol tov, selah.

Amen, He who has bestowed goodness upon you, may He bestow every goodness upon you forever.

Jewish law and birth—induction, cesarean section and eating your placenta—what's kosher?

There are a few things that happen during childbirth that trigger some Jewish law questions—the first of which is inducing labor. The rabbis say that God, in His wisdom, knows the best time for a baby to be born, and therefore we should not intervene unnecessarily. One of the great Rabbis, Rabbi Yohanan, explains that childbirth is one of the things in this world that only God has the key to. In addition, since childbirth is a potentially life-threatening situation, we should not bring it on earlier than necessary.

Jewish law stipulates that we should not intervene with the labor process unless there is an extreme risk for either mother or baby. The Jewish doulas I spoke with explain that this is an example where Jewish tradition can actually be more mother centered (as opposed to doctor or hospital centered) than our modern medical system. This would mean that scheduling a C-section for convenience, for example, would be against the spirit of the law. However, if your doctor advises an induction or cesarean, then Jewish law supports following their decision.

And in answer to a very common question about Jewish law when it comes to labor and delivery, let's get this one out of the way—YES, you can give birth on Shabbat! Of course, if it's God's will for the baby to be born at a certain time, then that is the time it will be! Because labor and delivery are life threatening situations, the mom's and baby's health are prioritized above all else.

And now the question you've all be waiting for: Is eating the placenta kosher?!

Well…it's debatable. According to some rabbis it is permissible by Jewish law; however the placenta eaten as food is not kosher. If you dry it and encapsulate it instead (which is how many women ingest it), it is no longer considered food. It is *d'var chadash*, something new, and therefore it can be declared medicine. There. It **is** kosher! In the same way, Jewish law permits us to take vitamins originally derived from oysters (an unkosher animal). If you are concerned about the kashrut status of your placenta, though, I'd encourage you to consult your own rabbi.

Fourth Trimester / Newborn

13.

Healing, Finding the New You and Postpartum Health

Look, just as time isn't inside clocks
love isn't inside bodies:
bodies only tell the love.
　　　—Yehuda Amichai

Although poetry is written to be interpreted and reimagined by the reader—intentionally to be personalized and experienced—I wonder if the famous Jewish poet Yehuda Amichai was possibly thinking about motherhood when he wrote that one. The experience of postpartum recovery is a lesson in just how much your body manifests the love you have for your new baby. Although it can be painful and exhausting, it's important to accept and acknowledge that giving yourself time to heal from such a tremendous change is necessary.

It takes nine months of biological changes to make a baby, and then, often very dramatically and suddenly, your body goes through one of the most epic physical experiences known to man (or really woman!) during labor and delivery. Think of it as a physical expression of the emotional change that occurs when you become a mom. Yesterday it was just you. Today you are a mother; you've created life. It's going to take some time for your body to stop telling you that 24/7.

Have you ever seen an elephant give birth? (For all those counting, yes this is the second time I've mentioned elephants and pregnancy in this book. Good memory! Just like an elephant. 🐘 ☺)If you have, you've witnessed one of the most miraculous things in nature. After dropping to the ground a few frightening feet from the mother's womb, the baby lands on some soft brush and the mom starts trumpeting to announce the arrival of her little one. Almost immediately she is surrounded by her herd, all rushing right in to protect the vulnerable baby and mom and investigate to make sure all is well. It's honestly breathtaking and heartwarming to witness. But, when I saw this spectacle of nature for the first time (on YouTube that is, unfortunately not in the actual Serengeti), it did leave me a bit sad. These creatures had figured out something we humans still have not—the art of community support for new moms.

Birth takes its toll on your body and your mind. It's OK to reach out to your tribe at this time. In fact, as any elephant will tell you, it's perfectly natural. I gave birth to one of the most easygoing babies who was honestly a little delight as a newborn, and I still struggled enormously with the "fourth trimester," as it's rightfully now called. The use of the term fourth trimester (the three or so months after giving birth) has really grown in popularity lately as mothers share the honest truth about the postpartum experience.

Hashtags like #stopcensoringmotherhood #rawmotherhood and #4thtrimesterbodies are popping up all over Twitter and Instagram as women campaign for a better understanding of the realities of the postpartum experience. For many women, recovering from birth is nothing like a fairy tale where you bounce back right out of the hospital. The physical pain from giving birth vaginally or having a C-section coupled with the enormous emotional toll of exhaustion and hormones balancing out is what makes any and every mom a **super** mom from day one!

Many women have very positive postpartum experiences and many recover easily and relatively quickly. It can be an enjoyable time of cocooned newborn cuddle sessions and sleepy early baby days. I heard many wonderful stories about how the first days with a newborn were the happiest of a mother's life. I know I felt that way. I was just surprised by the unexpectedness of the reality of those days and frustrated that no one had told me!

After my baby was born I hardly focused on my own self-care and healing. I was totally enamored of my son and spent all my attention on him. Even with the best of intentions and the easiest of births, it's important to set time aside for yourself, to heal. A lot of people ask me what my best advice is for new moms, and I like to say—lower your expectations (of yourself). After you've had a baby it can take a really long time to get your strength back, to get your body back (not only from pregnancy but from the grips of late night nursing and all day rocking!). It can be deeply fulfilling to take on the role of motherhood; but it's also deeply exhausting.

I had a particularly long and difficult recovery after giving birth, and was really surprised that I wasn't able to jump right back into my usual routine after the baby was born. I expected labor and delivery to be painful, but it seemed like no one spoke about postpartum as anything other than bliss. I wanted to just bask in the loving glow of a newborn baby, and genuinely had no idea that I would need to spend almost as much time and attention on my own body and healing as on the baby.

Your doctor may tell you not to lift heavy objects (especially after a C-section) and not to climb stairs or go on long walks, depending on whether you've had stitches or still have some bleeding. Many women ignore this advice and end up having longer recovery periods because of it. I was really curious though; why do women ignore self-care so often? Are you one of those women?

Katie, one of the moms I interviewed for this book, echoed this same sense of frustration that no one had told her how hard postpartum recovery would be and she wasn't prepared for what to expect. She told me that as a middle school teacher, once her students knew she was pregnant, "they were constantly telling me to sit down, to stop picking up pencils that had fallen on the floor, to stop putting up bulletin boards by myself." During her pregnancy she really appreciated this constant reminder that her growing baby needed her strength and energy. Then when her baby was born, she "forgot this advice and ended up really stressing my body postpartum. I tried to get back to normal way too quickly and ended up prolonging my recovery—my milk supply suffered temporarily and I had recurring bleeding. I didn't have my yoga teacher and my students there telling me to chill out! I should have kept them in my head!"

Moms-to-be spend so much mental energy preparing for *baby* that preparing for *me* often gets overlooked. Many women find this to be true to varying degrees. The most helpful mindset is to prepare for a few weeks of healing and recovery as your body heals. One of the most difficult realities of this is that many women are unaware of how common postpartum depression is and don't know what warning signs to watch for. When you think about it, why is your doctor mandated to ask you about your mental health after having a baby; shouldn't a woman know she's depressed? Amazingly, no! She can be so wrapped up in the to-do list of new motherhood and the exhaustion of newborn care that she may not even realize it.

Judaism and the art of healing

Judaism is all about living in the here and now. It's not about getting to heaven or the world to come, but living life to the fullest right here and right now. To be joyous and to create joy is a mitzvah; it's a mitzvah to dance at someone's wedding and to eat a delicious meal after a bris. One of the highest mitzvahs is to visit the sick and to care for them. Judaism places enormous emphasis on taking care of one of another and the community.

In this way Jewish community and culture is designed to be there for one another's ups and downs. In an article titled "The Heart of Jewish Joy,'" my childhood rabbi, Rabbi Ed Feinstein, Senior Rabbi of Valley Beth Shalom Synagogue in Encino, California, describes the very Jewish notion of seeking out light in times of darkness, and of turning toward Judaism to seek comfort and community. Let's face it: the Jewish people have been through **a lot**. There has been large-scale suffering that our entire people experienced, as well as small-scale suffering that every human life knows.

He said, "Who knows the world's darkness and brokenness better than we do? But standing before light and darkness, blessing and curse, life and death, we choose life. It may be the most difficult mitzvah in the Torah to fulfill. But we choose life. That is the heart of Jewish joy."

Judaism has a rich tradition of caring for new mothers and stipulates in both Jewish law and cultural history that new moms need to be cared for. Judaism places exceptionally high importance on a mother's recovery. Women are exempt from "time-bound" mitzvot (religious obligations that are required to be performed at specific times of the day) in order for them to be able to prioritize their families and family obligations. A pregnant and breastfeeding woman is also exempt from requirements like fasting during holidays like Yom Kippur.

Jewish law specifically mentions a time period of healing for a new mom. After giving birth and for the next weeks she is considered *niddah*—a status similar to having her period, and she should not have sex during that time.

I have written a lot about healing and recovery after birth, and in my work I advocate reaching out, speaking up and getting help. The physical and hormonal changes of pregnancy are enormous, and unlike anything else. It is **normal** to feel **not-normal**. There is no benefit to suffering silently.

Joel Kushner, director of the Kalsman Institute on Judaism and Health spoke to me about the rich tradition within Judaism for compassionate care. Part of the work of the Kalsman Institute is to bring issues like postpartum care into the light, because they are not just "women's issues"—they affect the entire community. These stigmas often delay care and diagnosis.

Jewish organizations like the Kalsman Institute are at the forefront of starting conversations with Jewish community leaders about maternal mental health issues. One in 4 women will experience a mental health concern after giving birth, and Jewish women are no exception. The core tradition of relieving women from the obligation of mitzvot after giving birth is a tradition that does not always translate into the modern world. Some women are expected to continue working and taking care of their homes and families just as they had before their child was born.

Support from your partner, family and community are an essential component of healing for a new mom. Rabbi Jaclyn Cohen of Temple Isaiah in West Los Angele says there's often a misperception about the human body and the experience of giving birth. She says people fundamentally don't understand that a new mom cannot just resume her normal routine after giving birth; in fact, pushing yourself too hard is harmful to the healing process.

This is one of the aspects of Jewish community, *kehila* in Hebrew, that can be especially helpful to those in their most vulnerable times in life. Synagogues will often arrange a "meal train" for new moms so that community members can sign up to bring meals and help out the family, in the same way they do when someone is sick.

Take these ancient customs as further confirmation that a new mom's role is self-care and care for her baby—not care for the laundry or the dishes. The Jewish community and her family need to nurture and love her first.

Meg is a mom who comes from a Chinese cultural background and is married to a Jewish man. She told me about all the Chinese customs she observed after having her babies. Following traditional Chinese custom and superstition, she was not allowed to leave the house with wet hair for one month after giving birth, and she was discouraged from washing her hair for the first month as well. She explained that Chinese customs have components of superstition and ancient beliefs about health and balance—the yin and yang. She also was prohibited from carrying heavy things and even from walking on tip toes while pregnant!

From an intermarried perspective she had to take into account both the Chinese and Jewish customs and faiths from her and her husband's family history. These cultural practices, as exhaustive as they may seem, are designed to help a mom heal. Before the days of Instagram, hundreds and thousands of years before the modern demands of a woman to be all and do all, religion and culture across the world sought to protect new moms during what they saw as the obvious and necessary period of healing.

One organization centered on Jewish women's wellness that may also be helpful for you is called At The Well. They support Well Circles, which are monthly meetup groups that get together around Rosh Chodesh each month. Rosh Chodesh is the first day of each Jewish month (based on the lunar calendar), and is a traditional holiday that is connected to the female side of us.

With the Hebrew calendar as a bedrock, At The Well shares their take on ritual through a "wellness lens." I spoke with Sarah Waxman, Director of the organization. She shared with me how women coming together and forming their own grassroots networks can be an enormously healing experience. When a new Well Circle commits to meeting each month, the women find a new sense of *kehila* or community, which can be especially helpful for new moms who very often feel isolated. Because these groups sit together and talk, it's also a chance for new moms to use an intellectual side of their brain that may be ignored during the daily grind of newborn care and late-night feedings.

One of Sarah's goals is to help women feel "nourished" Jewishly, and she started At The Well as the first organization to support women through Rosh Chodesh in this way. The sense of belonging and female friendship is such a helpful and necessary support system for new moms, Check on their website and Instagram to see if joining or starting a Well Circle is right for you. You can also follow them on Instagram *@AtTheWellproject* for daily inspiration.

Unfortunately and quite unexpectedly for many women, the postpartum experience can be a lonely and painful experience. I hope that your faith and community can be there for you if this is the reality you face when bringing home a new baby.

Recovery from a traumatic birth experience

I left the hospital in tears, and it was raining, so things were just... dramatic. But I was just **so grateful** to have made it out of there with a happy and healthy baby. I knew I had suffered in the process but ultimately that maternal instinct of "I would fight a bear to protect this baby" kicked in and I just felt total relief at being able to bring my baby home. I think that because I was so focused on the health of my baby, I didn't spend any mental energy grappling with what had just happened to my body. I'll spare you the gory details, but I left the hospital with a fracture in my spine, a catheter in my urethra (at least I think that's where they put it; I had no idea), and stitches in my you-know-where. OK, I guess I left a few gory details in!

I knew something was wrong but I was told repeatedly by the nursing staff that everyone is in pain after having a baby, and to just deal with it. Most women are fortunate not to suffer this kind of abuse, but I believed them—even though every nerve in my body (especially the ones down below) were screaming that this wasn't right.

Coming home with a baby who wouldn't latch on and a bris to plan meant I spent the next week on pure adrenaline. I couldn't walk down the stairs in my home but I didn't even call my doctor to let him know this. I just repeated the nurses' mantra to myself: everyone is in pain after giving birth; get over it. A lot of research has been done on trauma survivors and a lot of women experience a "freeze" mentality where their mind almost escapes their body to escape their pain. And as a result, they don't deal with it.

I didn't even get an X-ray of my spine until five months after my son was born. When I heard the result from the doctor that there had been a small fracture in one of my vertebrae, I burst out in tears. In a strange way it was like receiving a diagnosis for something I had already recovered from, because at that point I could walk just fine and was just in that residual aching pain stage. But I was shaking and in tears in his office because I felt such immense sympathy for myself; how had I let my own health and care be ignored for so long? I didn't research post-traumatic stress from birth for many more months; but after doing so, I realized how common my story is.

If you feel unhappy with your birth experience—if you feel like something went wrong—speak up and get help. Talk to your doctor, talk to a therapist, and connect with others online or in person who have had the same experience. Don't be surprised or disappointed if the first person you approach doesn't listen. I had an army of the best trained nurses in the nation ignoring me; just keep speaking up. The mental stress can take time to reveal itself and may come out in unexpected ways. Even if you have no lasting impact from a negative experience, you deserve to be heard and validated.

Who am I now that I'm a mom?

The hardest moment for me after my son was born happened the second day after we had come home from the hospital. Everything was **just so hard**. Just getting up to pee was a struggle. Nothing was how I imagined new mom bliss to be. My house was the opposite of the Pinterest ideal I had spent months scrolling through; there was no gorgeous nursery for me to take photos of in my floral robe with a fresh blowout.

Instead, there were boxes **everywhere** and I was in too much pain to get out of bed, let alone get a blowout. My husband and I were sitting at the dinner table and eating deli carryout that our family had brought over. I remember it so well because we ate only deli sliced turkey, rye bread, kettle cooked chips and salad that his grandma had brought over that entire week; honestly, it was pretty good. But it wasn't my normal cooking and the house and everything in it just seemed so different already. My dogs were with a dog sitter, there were baby swings and diapers all over the place, and it just all felt so strange.

I missed my life, my body, my health. That was really the hardest moment and it was just the beginning, because when you give birth everything changes **in an instant**. You have nine months to prepare for something you can't prepare for, for an experience you have little control over, and for a new family member you've invited in but have no idea what the heck they will be like. It's really incomparable to any other life experience.

This was just a mini moment of baby blues for me and I very thankfully didn't suffer postpartum depression as so many women do; but it was the profound shift that was so emotional and shocking to me. I wanted to be a mom. I wanted nothing more, but it was still hard to make peace with the fact that motherhood wasn't going to be on my terms just yet—everything was for this little baby and his needs. I breastfed him and pumped every 2 hours in those first 10 days. Which meant feeding for a half hour, resting for a half hour, pumping for a half hour and resting again for a half hour. It was honestly insane. But I fought for it, for my baby, for the motherhood I wanted. In that process every other part of my identity disappeared.

But they came back. The dogs, the ability to cook my own meals, the feeling that it was all going to be OK. Slowly but surely they all returned and with them so did my sense of who I was in all of this. The newborn days are a time warp and a twilight zone, but they're not forever. I learned to fine tune my identity and that I wasn't *just* a mom (even though those early days felt that way), but it took time to figure it all out again.

There's an ancient Jewish story that perfectly characterizes the feeling of being a new mom. The story is about a king—well not just a king—**the** king, the wise King Solomon. One day he asked his servant to bring him a special ring, a ring with a magical power. He described the ring in this way: when a happy person wears it he becomes sad, and when a sad person wears it he becomes happy. His faithful servant Benaiah answered him, "If it exists your majesty, I will find it for you." Benaiah and his soldiers searched far and wide and he feared they would come up empty-handed.

They found the most expensive and most beautiful rings with sparkling jewels from across the world, but not the magic ring. Benaiah asked a simple silversmith if he knew of the magic ring and where it could be found. To Benaiah's surprise the silversmith presented it to him, a simple ring, but when he read the words inscribed in it he understood that he had found what the king asked of him. When Benaiah returned to the king and presented the ring to him, legend has it he cried. The great men and women in the king's court watched in silence, what could make this great king cry? He read to them what was written within: *Gam Zeh Ya'avor—This Too Shall Pass*.

I held tightly to this mantra during the longest nights and most exhausting days of new motherhood. I always laughed to myself and thought, I won't be holding him in my arms and singing him lullabies when he goes off to college, and I'm sure I'll wish I had held him just a bit longer, that I had just one more night to gently pull my fingers through his soft hair and look down at his little baby face. So when his cries woke me at three in the morning and my eyes literally hurt from exhaustion begging to be closed, I thought, "this too shall pass," and found great comfort in it. Millions of women before me and after me have survived this, and I can, too.

I also learned to ask for help, which I hate doing! In my mind I wanted to excel at motherhood and this identity ideal meant I tried to do it all and all by myself. The real moms I interviewed for this book shared that they too had learnt this lesson the hard way. There's no award for breastfeeding and there's no prize for never resorting to Sesame Street when it's 5:00 pm and you just need to get dinner on the table; or better yet, sit on the toilet for 5 minutes, or even— miracle of miracles—have an actual shower. Don't let trying to be the "perfect" mom stop you from being a happy and healthy person.

Can you be a stay-at-home-mom feminist?
Here's some Mama motivation

As your little newborn becomes a baby and then a toddler, your own identity grows and changes as well. What does it mean for your career and your interests?

I attended an event at Sixth & I Synagogue in Washington, D.C., where author Deb Perelmen of the website Smitten Kitchen came to talk and do a live Q&A. A very inquisitive young female audience member asked her if her devotion to cooking was a little antiquated, a little unprogressive? And this comment really shook me. What if you love doing something (like cooking, or cleaning or even... not working outside the home) that generations of women fought against having to do? Can a stay-at-home-mom also be a role model for women?

From the mothers I interviewed who shared thoughts on this notion of guilt, I was further convinced that no one can have it *all*, so you have to create the life you want for yourself and your family. If you find joy, passion and empowerment in the kitchen, then it is your domain to rule. If you find it in the boardroom, then rock it there. Don't let anyone else's expectation of where you've been dictate where you're going.

As my therapist likes to remind me, moms are really good at feeling guilty. Whatever flavor guilt you may be experiencing, women are exceptionally talented at seeing themselves negatively— no matter how much effort and love and skill they put into to what they're doing. There's a Yiddish saying that, "You can't dance at two weddings"—*Mit eyn tokhes ken men nit tantsn af tsvey khasen*—and the truth of being in two places at once and "leaning in" everywhere all the time is just not possible. As a result a lot of women feel immense guilt when they either go back to work or step back from their careers to stay home.

I walked away from a six-figure income in a career I loved and had built over 10 years to spend more time with my son. Even more shocking than that, I walked away from the societal expectation that an educated, talented young woman should succeed in business because she could. A seat at the boardroom table is what women have been fighting for, and it seemed like it was my time to fight for it. But in the prime of my career, I walked away.

It was my choice, and I was lucky enough to have the financial capability to do so. I struggled with the guilt over my decision; was I a bad role model? Had I wasted my education? I justified my choice in saying that I was starting my YouTube Channel, writing this book and scraping together a way to be the boss of my own business. But many women don't have a cover story, and they just embrace the fact that motherhood is calling them in a strong way away from the office. I consider myself a full circle feminist. I wasn't forced to stay home because of a glass ceiling; I chose to change how I spent my days in a move of self-empowerment. For me I knew I would regret the time I was missing away from my son by being in an office setting, and that was something I could never get back.

Personally I chose to stop working 40 hours a week in an office setting when my older son turned two and it felt like the most empowering and brave decision I'd made. Going to college and then business school and then embarking on a high-stress high-reward career in television production felt like easy decisions to me. I followed a predictable path and worked hard to achieve my goals. When motherhood came along, I was really taken aback by how desperately I wanted to be a full-time mom.

Was I a failed feminist? A product of a generation raised on "Yes you can," only to say "No thank you, I'd rather not"? I felt judged and like an outsider among my peer group who almost all had nannies and went back to high-powered positions in the workforce. In my heart though, I knew that no career would be fulfilling to me when every day in the office my thoughts always drifted to my son. I was determined to continue to pursue my creative writing and my YouTube channel, so I did have part-time work to take on when I did eventually leave my full-time job. But it was still a difficult and emotional decision. I left behind a team and boss I loved and a career that I had devoted a decade to building. I felt guilty about the cost (both time and financially) of the education I had received and of the years of training and grinding I had spent to get to where I was in my field.

At the same time many women told me they feel guilty about the long hours they spend at the office and that they're not home with their children all day. So is this whole motherhood thing rigged? When you have a child, the reality is that work will never be the same; as a primary caregiver there will now always be someone to think about and care for. And when you have a career, motherhood is never the same because you'll always have a meeting you need to leave early from and a project you can't take on because you have a sick kid at home.

Being a "good mom" and a "good employee" isn't about a tally of hours spent with your child or your computer. A lot of women I spoke with carry a lot of guilt that physically and emotionally weighs them down, and it isn't serving them or helping them in any way. Letting go of the guilt is the best way to live in the moment and be present wherever you spend your day. And if you choose to make a monumental life change, as Ryan Seacrest once said on his radio show on KIIS FM in Los Angeles, "Never be a prisoner of your past. It was just a lesson, not a life sentence."

Postpartum depression

While the postpartum experience can be a physically and emotionally intense time for everyone as your body heals and your hormones level out, there are some experiences that are not normal and should be treated by a medical professional. Before giving birth my husband and I both read up on the warning signs for postpartum depression. What really frightened me was that mothers don't always realize they have it, and often their partners need to step up and step in to help. So I wanted my husband to know what to look for and when to get help. Thankfully, while my postpartum experience was extremely challenging physically, I did not suffer from depression. However, there are many Jewish women who do. If you think you may be experiencing some of the symptoms of PPD, know that you are not the only Jewish mom to have gone through this and there are resources to help you.

Rabbi Jaclyn Cohen of Temple Isaiah in West Los Angeles, who contributed to this book, speaks openly and passionately about her experience with postpartum depression. She is one of the most vocal and inspirational voices in the Jewish community on this topic. She discusses how some of the expectations, pressures and assumptions mentioned earlier in this chapter contributed first to her mental state, but also to her not realizing how far down she had sunk. Her loved ones stepped in and she got the help she needed; she is better now and has enormous empathy for moms in a similar situation. She has many resources available on her website that I highly recommend if you are in the midst of a PPD diagnosis or think it is something you may be experiencing (jaclynfcohen.com).

Although Rabbi Cohen is a changemaker in the Jewish world because she speaks so openly about mental issues, it is not uncommon for Jewish people to seek help from their rabbis in their time of need. Your rabbi can be a strong part of your support system as you heal during this time and the synagogue can provide a network of services and connections for you and your family.

14.

Breastfeeding, Bottle Feeding... What's Kosher? Plus First Foods and Jewish First Foods

Humans have been feeding babies for hundreds of thousands of years, but there is still controversy over the best way to do it. With each generation there's a fresh debate over which method creates the healthiest and happiest mom and baby. In this chapter I want to share some ancient Jewish wisdom and perspective on breastfeeding. That's not to say that Judaism is against formula feeding; it's just that like much of Judaism, our customs were written down and entrenched in tradition long before relatively newer developments like formula even existed.

Like most Jewish law, rules on feeding a baby were codified centuries before women worked in office buildings 9-5 and before formula existed. While breastfeeding can be a beautiful and spiritual way to connect to your baby, some women find it exhausting, painful and sometimes altogether impossible. Many Jewish women supplement or substitute with formula. The most critical Jewish law is *picuach nefesh*, the commandment to place saving a life above all else. If you are struggling to breastfeed, know that the most important Jewish value is preserving the life of your baby.

I was very determined to breastfeed my son and did so until he was 18 months old. I had read before giving birth about the benefits of breastmilk and I knew it would be a sacrifice of my time and comfort to breastfeed exclusively, but it was just something I knew I did not want to compromise on. I had to hire a lactation consultant twice, and the first two weeks of my son's life consisted of round-the-clock nursing, pumping and syringe-feeding expressed milk, which resulted in never more than a two-hour-long sleep for either me or him.

Each mom knows what's important to them and what they won't compromise on; for me it was nursing. However, after those initial two weeks and the use of a nipple shield (a controversial little thing in the breastfeeding community!) I honestly found breastfeeding very easy and soothing. I was lucky and enjoyed it; it never felt like much of a burden to me and I believe that was a combination of having a relatively easy time of it physically and being emotionally convinced of its benefits.

However, many of the Jewish moms I spoke with told me that breastfeeding was not something they could enjoy or maintain long after their babies were born. Many felt that being able to return to a sense of normalcy—whether that involved working or just sleeping—was more important to their overall health and happiness, which in turn was better for the baby.

While formula didn't exist in Biblical times, there are stories in the Torah of *nursemaids* or *wet nurses*—women brought in to nurse babies when their mothers couldn't. There are many famous stories of the importance of these women, such as Rachel's nursemaid Devorah, who plays an important role in her and Jacob's story.

Breastfeeding and Judaism, a divine and ancient practice

Judaism treats breastfeeding as a visceral example of where we can see miracles here on Earth. Jewish tradition compares a mother's ability to feed her baby to a divine experience—and if you've ever tried breastfeeding it sure can feel that way when you finally get the hang of it! Breastfeeding is a revered and exalted experience in Judaism.

Let's pause here for just a moment, because this is **huge**! For a religion whose text was largely written down by men centuries ago, there is still an emphasis on and acknowledgment of the sacred importance of a mother's role to care for her baby. This is a beautiful thing; as a modern woman who can sometimes be critical of the lack of equality or feminism in religion, I want to take a moment to celebrate this.

We hear about breastfeeding in the Torah, most famously in the story of Moses. When the Egyptian princess found baby Moses, he refused to nurse from an Egyptian nursemaid and a Jewish one was brought instead—who turned out to be his own mother, Yocheved. This is taken as especially meaningful, imbuing the idea that a mother's milk isn't just for the sake of nutrition. It is believed that Yocheved had an early influence on Moses; through nursing him she taught him kindness and compassion and a love for his people.

There are also many references to the Jewish people receiving God's words and love, comparing the experience to a baby receiving milk from her mother. This imagery appears throughout ancient Jewish texts. In the Book of Isaiah the Jewish people are living in exile and fear that God has abandoned them. In answer to their cries God promises to console the Jewish people like a mother comforting a son. God compares his love to a mother who has nursed her baby, saying that He could never forget his people just as a mother could never forget her child who nursed from her for so long.

Even more explicitly, rabbis compare the manna that the Israelites eat during their 40 years of wandering to the milk with which a mother feeds her child:

> The ensuing forty years of wandering in the desert could also be compared to the forty weeks of pregnancy in which babies gestate waiting for the Promised Land. Once they are free, they will survive on a single food source from their mother, breastmilk, in much the same way as the Israelites survived on manna in the wilderness. Just as with the breast, which changes to take on many tastes, so too the manna turned into whatever food they wanted. Just as with the breast, the baby suffers when s/he separates from it, so too Israel suffered when separating from the manna. –Rabbi Jeffrey Clopper

The story of Exodus itself has many links to the ideas of fertility and birth, rabbis compare the story of our people leaving Egypt and reaching the Promised Land as a birth experience in itself. We emerged from slavery as a free people and our journey through the desert to get there was a pregnancy of sorts. It took time for God to shape his people with his laws until they were ready for life in a free land. Aside from these poetic anologies there is also many specific references to elements of birth and laws regarding motherhood in the Torah.

The Talmud also explicitly discusses breastfeeding. The *Shulchan Aruch*, a code of Jewish law written in the fifteenth century, mentions a timeline for breastfeeding. The *Shulchan Aruch* specifies a minimum of two and a maximum of five years as a requirement for mothers to nurse their babies (*Even Haezer* 143:8, *Yore Deah* 81:7). Even Maimonides weighed in on the topic, recommending breastfeeding in his *Mishnah Torah Le Rambam*, compiled in the eleventh century. Jewish tradition also recommends beginning to breastfeed on the left side, closest to the mother's heart.

The Hebrew word for a nursing baby is *gamul*, which also has the same Hebrew root as the word *gomel*, which means to perform an act of kindness. Jewish text commentators say this connection implies that for a mother to nurse her child is an act of loving kindness.

Is breast milk kosher and is it OK to breastfeed in public?

Some people have asked me if breast milk itself is kosher, and indeed it is! It's even considered pareve—not meat (*flaishich*) or dairy (*milchik*). However, there are a lot of *kashrut* customs about how things appear, so you aren't likely to see observant families giving a baby breast milk from a bottle while they're eating meat—because it might give someone the impression that they were mixing meat and milk.

Many rabbis have weighed in on all sorts of minutiae: is breast milk from a non-Jewish mother kosher? What about milk from a

Jewish mother who doesn't keep kosher? Is expressed milk kosher to drink at any age? How long can a child breastfeed? I've decided to refrain from giving answers on these topics, because I believe that if you are observant enough to really be concerned about these questions you will turn to your rabbi for an answer! However, I do think it's important to share the basic foundation for Jewish thought on feeding babies. Breast milk is definitely kosher and in most modern and liberal communities it is not considered immodest to breastfeed in public.

The Conservative Movement in Judaism has even sanctioned breastfeeding in synagogue, as it is also legal to breastfeed in public in the United States. According to Rabbi Artson of the Jewish Theological Seminary, discouraging nursing in the sanctuary is "a mistaken idea of what *kavod hatzibur* [honoring the synagogue's dignity] is…There is no greater image of the love of God for humanity than a nursing mother, and no greater image for the way the Torah is lovingly transmitted from one generation to another than a nursing mother."

You're unlikely to see a mother nursing in an Orthodox synagogue because they would follow the tradition of staying home during this time; or for the sake of modesty, not nursing in public. Post-partum, all new mothers, including those who are nursing, are considered *meineket*, and retain this special status until the child is two years old. New mothers are exempt from certain *mitzvot* (commandments) such as fasting and being in synagogue.

Can you pump on Shabbat?

This is a very interesting question and it gets into some very detailed *halacha (*Jewish law). Strictly speaking, the answer is no; a woman should not use a breast pump or even hand express breast milk for the purpose of using it at another time. So it is against strict observance of Shabbat to pump into a bottle and store the breast milk.

However, there are two exceptions to this rule—one for the health of the mother and one for the health of the baby. If the mother is engorged or in pain from mastitis, for example, she is permitted to express milk on Shabbat, but she should not save it for use at a later time. If the infant cannot latch and needs to use a bottle, then the mother can express milk into the bottle for the baby. This may initially seem like a complicated and strict answer but the heart of the matter is this: as with all Jewish law, life and health are more important than anything else. That is an essential component of Judaism and of leading a Jewish life—act in a way that pursues life and health.

Is infant formula kosher?

Yes! There are many brands that are labeled kosher.

The sanctity and purity of food is a central component of Judaism and ancient dietary laws of *kashrut* were based on both the spiritual and physical health of the Jewish people. Many customs such hand washing and preparing meat helped Jewish people avoid disease. As Judaism evolves with modern times the health and well-being of the child is always paramount. Jewish tradition encourages mothers to listen to medical advice above all else; so if your doctor or your baby's pediatrician recommends including formula in their diet, then it's important to follow their instruction.

A quick note on Israeli baby food

When your baby starts on their solid food journey, you can ask your pediatrician about introducing peanut butter through an Israeli snack called Bamba. Not only is this stuff delicious (think of it as a peanut butter flavored puff snack), it's really easy for babies to eat and snack on the go. A study showed that children in Israel have a significantly lower rate of peanut allergies likely because they eat so much of it!

15.
What's a Jewish Nursery?
and other Jewish Baby Ideas

If you're anything like me, you probably have a never-ending list of baby preparations to get done before your due date. I know in my case it was a 10 tab Excel spreadsheet that kept me busy. I had a list of things to buy before the baby arrived (onesies, diapers, car seat, nipple cream); a list of things that needed to be done right after the baby arrived (calls to the insurance company, the pediatrician, the newborn photographer); a tab where I collected addresses for bris invites and thank you notes; a tab of baby name ideas (including an even longer one of names my husband and I had already vetoed)... the lists went on and on. In all honesty, planning for me is a way of passing the time before the big event, and it's one I enjoy. Aside from all this minutiae, there are bigger things to start thinking about. One of them is how to incorporate Jewish tradition, customs and values into your home and your life with the arrival of a new baby.

A Jewish nursery room for baby

Designing a nursery is a quintessential motherhood step that often begins on a Pinterest board and ends in a desperate midnight online search for a vintage car themed night light (just me?). Even if you're planning to keep it super simple, there is something so special about planning out what your child's bedroom will look like, knowing how many memories will soon take place there. While you're in the planning stages of even the most Instagram-worthy #nursery, there are many Jewish elements you can incorporate in the room. These items are often meaningful and personal and can hold a lot of sentimental value.

In my home we have a few very special items in my baby's room: a mezuzah we designed for him to match his room colors; a handmade piece of art with his Hebrew name from his by his aunt and uncle; and a stuffed toy Torah that we gave him as a Hanukkah gift. These pieces are some of my favorites in the room because they were made and given with love! Always planning ahead, we have a Hebrew letter puzzle and Jewish books ready for our son as he grows up.

Rachel, one of the Jewish moms I interviewed for this book, had lots of ideas about adding Jewish components to a nursery. She had each of her children's Hebrew names made into beautiful artwork for their rooms, and hung a personalized mezuzah on each of their doors. She also incorporated Hebrew and Judaic kids' books into the nursery, and even purchased some Jewish themed toys like the KidKraft wooden holiday sets.

Shira, another mom I spoke with, told me that each of her first two children were gifted tzedakah boxes when they were born and that her two older girls will give their new baby sister one for her to keep.

There are so many beautiful traditions like these to start in your own family, so as you prep and plan and make lists, think about which of them you might like to include.

Why all the emphasis on this early introduction to Jewish customs? In the Torah we are directly told to teach—diligently teach—our children to love God and to keep His words, the words of Torah, in our hearts and in theirs: "And you shall teach them to your sons" (Deuteronomy 11:19)

Whatever your beliefs regarding God and the Bible are, the core value here is spiritual education. Being a good Jewish mom doesn't mean making challah from scratch every Friday; it means teaching children to love this world, instilling in them a lifelong love of learning and a love of their faith.

Part of the way we start along that journey as Jewish parents is by incorporating touches of Judaism in their space, at their eye level, so that it becomes a physical part of their world.

A mezuzah for the nursery

There's really just one thing that, according to Jewish law, you need to have in your baby's nursery room (well, just outside their room, really), and that's a mezuzah. It's Jewish custom to hang a mezuzah on the doorframe or doorpost of all the rooms in your home, and the baby's room is no exception. There are so many beautiful mezuzot out there and you can even find one to match the theme or decor of your nursery.

Jews put the words of the *Shema* and *Veahavta* prayers inscribed on a scroll inside every mezuzah on every entrance to a living space in their home because God instructed us in the Torah to remember these specific words and to live by them. These words tell us to love God and to teach this love to our children. So some would say that the mezuzah on the door to your child's bedroom is, therefore, the most important one in the home.

Here is a translation of the verses written on the scroll of the mezuzah:

"Hear, O Israel! God is our God, God alone.

You shall love God your God with all your heart and with all your soul and with all your might.

Take to heart these instructions with which I charge you this day.

Impress them upon your children. Recite them when you stay at home and when you are away, when you lie down and when you get up.

Bind them as a sign on your hand and let them serve as a symbol on your forehead; inscribe them on the doorposts of your house and on your gates.

If, then, you obey the commandments that I enjoin upon you this day, loving God your God and serving Him with all your heart and soul, I will grant the rain for your land in season, the early rain and the late. You shall gather in your new grain and wine and oil— I will also provide grass in the fields for your cattle—and thus you shall eat your fill.

Take care not to be lured away to serve other gods and bow to them.

For God's anger will flare up against you, and He will shut up the skies so that there will be no rain and the ground will not yield its produce; and you will soon perish from the good land that God is assigning to you.

Therefore impress these My words upon your very heart: bind them as a sign on your hand and let them serve as a symbol on your forehead, and teach them to your children—reciting them when you stay at home and when you are away, when you lie down and when you get up; and inscribe them on the doorposts of your house and on your gates— to the end that you and your children may endure, in the land that God swore to your fathers to assign to them, as long as there is a heaven over the earth."

—Deuteronomy 6:4-9 and Deuteronomy 11:13-21

You can purchase mezuzot personalized with the baby's name or with cute nursery designs on them. In our home we have one that says Max (our son's name) and has little cars painted on it to match his car themed playroom (it was actually a very thoughtful gift we inherited when he was born!). You can find mezuzot online and at your local Judaica store or synagogue gift shop. This is also a lovely gift idea for someone who has recently had a baby or moved into a new house!

It is important to note that for a mezuzah to be considered kosher, the parchment inside, the *klaf,* must be written by hand, just like the Torah itself. The parchment must come from a kosher animal and the scribe who writes on the scroll must do so carefully without making any mistakes. These rolls can be expensive because of the labor and skill required to make them.

Hanging up the mezuzah on the doorframe of your baby's room

is really simple. All you need is the mezuzah and *klaf* (the small parchment roll inside the mezuzah), and nails or a strong adhesive to secure it to the wall. The mounting is kosher so long as it is "well affixed" so nails are not required. It is traditional **not** to use a clear glass or Lucite mezuzah (or rather mezuzah case) on a bedroom or bathroom, so you shouldn't be able to see the scroll inside a nursery mezuzah.

How to put up a mezuzah in the nursery

Here are the steps to hang up a mezuzah the kosher way. I also have a YouTube video on my MyJewishMommyLife channel about this if you would like to see a demonstration (just search YouTube for "MyJewishMommyLife mezuzah").

It is also a lovely tradition to have the baby with you when you put up the mezuzah on his doorway. You might want to do this when you transition your child from your room to their own room. You could take this time to offer a special prayer to him and wish him a long life of happiness as he grows up in that room. If your child is a bit older, you can explain the mitzvah and include him in the process; you could even let him pick out his own mezuzah.

Step 1: Mark the spot on the doorpost where you are going to place the mezuzah. It should be about two thirds of the way up the doorway on the right-hand side as you walk into the room.

Step 2: Say the prayer! There is a simple prayer for hanging up a mezuzah. There are just two words at the end that are special; the beginning of the prayer follows the same format as all Jewish prayers:

בָּרוּךְ אַתָּה אַדֹנָי אֱלֹהֵינוּ מֶלֶךְ הָעוֹלָם,
אֲשֶׁר קִדְּשָׁנוּ בְּמִצְוֹתָיו וְצִוָּנוּ לִקְבּוֹעַ מְזוּזָה

Barukh atah Adonai Eloheinu melekh ha'olam,
asher kideshanu bemitzvotav vetzivanu liqboa' mezuzah.

Blessed are You, Lord our God, King of the Universe, Who sanctified us with His mitzvot, and commanded us to affix a mezuzah.

Step 3: Nail in the top of the mezuzah. It should be placed in a slanted direction with the top of the mezuzah facing in toward the room.

Step 4: Nail in the bottom of the mezuzah. The mezuzah should rest at about a 30 to 45 degree angle toward the inside of the room.

That's it! It is customary to kiss the mezuzah with your hand when you walk into the room, and it is believed to bring good luck.

Jewish music for children & Jewish/Israeli nursery rhymes

When my baby was born I couldn't wait to participate in all the Jewish family activities I had been eyeing from afar, and remembered being a part of when I was little. From Tot Shabbats to Shabbat story times, synagogues and Jewish Community Centers have so many options for being a part of Jewish life when you have little ones. I soon realized, though, that these activities are not really for the newborn stage. I felt a little lost and disappointed because I didn't know how to do anything "Jewish" with my baby. The first Jewish activity my son and I found together was random, and it turned out to be Jewish baby music!

Baby music is crazy weird; babies actually prefer it to adult music and I'm really not sure why that is. I find this so bizarre but it's not a fluke, there's something about children's music that children actually like and adults usually don't. Maybe this makes sense to most of you; I personally didn't believe it and thought it was a bunch of mumbo jumbo. But I found out the hard way (with my baby screaming in the back seat of the car) that the baby wanted to listen to baby music, usually on repeat. So we compromised. I like Jewish music; I like that there are Hebrew words and Jewish values woven into the beautiful melodies, so I downloaded Jewish lullabies and Jewish children's songs to listen to. And just like that we had started our first Jewish family tradition!

I figured out that music is actually one of the first activities you can share with your baby and one of the best ways to learn and bond. I sing songs to my baby before bed and we listen to them in the car. Now he's old enough to ask Google to play "Bim Bam" for himself and I'm pretty sure I've heard it over 100,000 times by this point (Is there a loyalty club for that sort of thing?). We're not *religious* (pun intended) about it, but especially on Fridays as we get ready for Shabbat or around holiday times, I just love incorporating this spiritual and festive music into our daily routine.

Here are my favorite children's music artists:

❏ Cindy Paley Aboody
❏ Isaac Zones
❏ Craig Taubman
❏ Rick Recht
❏ Melita Silberstein
❏ Robbo

And if you're new to the Jewish music scene, check out pjlibraryradio.com, where you can listen to tons of Jewish kids music for free!

Jewish toys and nursery decor

I invite you to do a walking tour of your home; how many items do you come across that are Jewish? In my home you'll find a mezuzah as you enter through the front hall doorway; some beautiful Judaic holiday art behind glass shelves in my kitchen; our wedding Ketubah hanging up on the wall in our bedroom. At first glance it might seem that my home is filled with Jewish items. But now go on a tour at the height of a toddler, or even crawl around to get a baby's perspective. Are any of the items ones they can touch or even see? Most likely not.

This is why investing in some Jewish kids' items is really worthwhile for little ones. Being able to see and touch objects is an important component of learning. One of the least expensive first things you can buy for your child is a Jewish book. There are so many board books about Shabbat, Jewish values and Jewish holidays that it would be easy to fill their first bookshelves with them. There is also a free program called PJ Library (PJLibrary.org) for Jewish children six months old and up.

Each month they'll receive a new Jewish book through PJ Library for free in the mail, tailored to their age and the season of the year. My family already has quite a little collection on our PJ Library shelf, and it's very exciting to see what new book will arrive each month in the mail. PJ Library also has books available for parents, plus many educational resources on their website. The books cover a variety of Jewish related topics like the holidays, Israel and Jewish values and are written specifically to be age-appropriate. The organization receives generous funding to support early childhood literacy and children's first Jewish education.

Play is also an essential element of a child's growth and development. There are lovely Jewish themed wooden toys available, including Shabbat and holiday pretend food sets, Hebrew letter puzzles and lots of holiday-related items like Hanukkah dreidels for kids. I like to mix these items in with my son's other toys, and we talk about them and their meaning as we play with them. In this way they become familiar and fun to play with without a formal lesson. As Mr. Rogers says, sometimes the best way to learn is when things are caught rather than taught!

The best places to find Jewish toys might be your local Judaica gift shop at a synagogue nearby, and of course online - Amazon has almost everything these days! You can find 'stuffed' torahs (think stuffed animal but in the shape of a friendly Torah!), Hebrew letter blocks and puzzles and lots of holiday themed playsets, like wooden Shabbat candlesticks and Shabbat food like challah. Hanukkah items are also very popular with dreidels, gelt and Hannukiahs designed for all different ages.

My personal list of the best Jewish books for kids

The Carp in the Bathtub by Barbara Cohen

This is truly a classic. It's very old and, dare I say, old-fashioned even—but it paints a picture of traditional Jewish life we don't see much of anymore. The story revolves around a fish in a bathtub that's going to be served for the Passover Seder. Oy!

Stories for Children: A Collection by Isaac Bashevis Singer

Singer is one of the most famous Jewish authors and his writing is the ultimate classic. Find a good collection of his short stories and you will be set. They have many Yiddish words and values woven into them and tell of families in European shtetl life from which much Jewish culture we know of today originates.

All-of-a-Kind Family by Sydney Taylor

A famous series of books about a large Jewish family living in New York City in the early twentieth century. This was one of the first series of its kind about a Jewish family and was my personal all-time favorite growing up!

Shabbat is Coming! by Tracy Newman

We have this book and I think just about every one written for each of the Jewish holidays. They are short rhyming poem board books for little ones that highlight the celebration and joy of Jewish holidays.

I Dissent by Debbie Levy

A picture book sharing the life of Supreme Court Justice extraordinaire, the notorious RBG. Ruth Bader Ginsburg was one of the few women to become a Supreme Court Justice and was also Jewish.

Adding a blessing: making bedtime a Jewish experience

Bedtime, a tranquil moment of day full of soft lullabies and beautiful story book reading snuggled up quietly together. Until you have a toddler; then it's mostly running around the house naked, requests for one more story and another glass of milk, and full-blown tantrums when a stuffed animal you're fairly certain never existed can't be found.

But in all seriousness, bedtime offers parents a unique opportunity to send their child off to sleep feeling safe and loved. Bedtime is all about routine; figuring out a routine that works for your child is the best way to create healthy sleeping habits. In my home, that routine starts with bedtime, followed by two stories in the rocking chair, "blast off" into the crib, and two more stories in the crib. Then we sing the Shema prayer, turn off the lights and say "Love you, laila tov." That's how it *usually* goes; other nights it's the chaos described in the first paragraph. #toddlermomlife)

Bedtime is usually one of the few times of the day when your child is quiet and calm and you can talk to them about the day they've had, be introspective and grateful for what you've experienced and shared together. Sharing thoughts and feelings of gratitude is an essential Jewish value. You can also talk about what you'd like for the day ahead.

Most babies and toddlers fall into this simple bedtime routine: *bath, books, bedtime.* I like to add a fourth B to the mix—*blessing.*

The Shema prayer is a traditional bedtime prayer; it is customary in Judaism for everyone to recite it before bed. Here are the words in Hebrew, English and transliteration of the prayer.

שְׁמַע יִשְׂרָאֵל אֲדֹנָי אֱלֹהֵינוּ אֲדֹנָי אֶחָד

Sh'ma Yis-ra-eil, A-do-nai E-lo-hei-nu, A-do-nai E-chad.

Hear, Oh Israel the Lord our God; the Lord is one.

There is actually a longer version of the Shema prayer that is reserved especially for bedtime, called the *Kriat Shema al Hamitah* (in Hebrew *mitah* means bed). This tradition dates back to the time of the Talmud when Rabbi Yehoshua ben Levi said that it should be recited before we fall asleep. The Torah itself also directly mentions the commandment to recite the Shema, "when you lie down and when you get up" (Deuteronomy 6:7). The longer bedtime Shema is composed of a few different lines of prayer. I was surprised when researching this prayer that one of the lines in the prayer comes from the same line in the Adon Olam, as translated here by The Rabbinical Assembly for Siddur Sim Shalom, "I place my spirit in His care, when I wake and when I sleep. God is with me; I shall not fear." The Adon Olam prayer actually has some historic roots as a traditional bedtime prayer.

Here is the English translation of a shortened bedtime Shema for children from the Siddur Sim Shalom:

Hear, O Israel: the Lord our God, the Lord is One.
Praised is the Lord by day and praised by night,
praised when we lie down and praised when we rise up.
I place my spirit in His care, when I wake as when I sleep.
God is with me, I shall not fear, body and spirit in His keep.

As parents you can also add in your own thoughts, whether quietly in your head or out loud, thanking God for the blessing of the day you've just had, for a good night's sleep and for a new day ahead. Whether you choose to mention God or not, and whether you personally believe in a higher power, the point really is just to connect with your child and let them know that your thoughts are of them and of all good things for them.

Going to bed and being alone at night can be scary for a child—for anyone really—and hearing a word of blessing and love from you before you leave their room can be enormously comforting and calming.

Another lovely tradition is to sing the Modeh Ani morning prayer with your child when you wake up. Here is the translation and transliteration by the Artscroll siddur:

מוֹדֶה אֲנִי לְפָנֶיךָ מֶלֶךְ חַי וְקַיָּם,
שֶׁהֶחֱזַרְתָּ בִּי נִשְׁמָתִי בְּחֶמְלָה. רַבָּה אֱמוּנָתֶךָ.

Modeh anee lefanecha melech chai vekayam,
she-he-chezarta bee nishmatee b'chemla, raba emunatecha.

I give thanks before you, King living and eternal, for You have returned within me my soul with compassion; abundant is Your faithfulness.

Rachel, who shared her advice on raising Jewish children, told me that because one of her son's names is Benjamin (nicknamed B) this prayer took on an extra special meaning because she thought of him and his name when singing *"Bee" nishmatee* and felt she was personally thanking God who had woken her up and returned her son to her each morning.

There are so many things that come to mind when you sing a prayer to your child; it has a profound affect not just on your child but on you as well. It's rare that as a busy parent (is there such a thing as a not-busy parent?) that we also get the time for blessing and gratitude.

Shabbat with children

There are so many ways to make the Shabbat holiday fun for young children every week, from baking challah together to creating art projects and reading books to welcome in the Sabbath. I want to touch on just the very basic rituals you can incorporate from the very first Shabbat you experience together as a family.

The first way Shabbat may change when you have children is that there are specific Shabbat blessings to be recited for children on

Friday nights. This tradition hearkens back to the Biblical story of Jacob and his son Joseph. Before Jacob died he rewarded his son Joseph, who had always been faithful to him, with a special prayer. He also included Joseph's two sons Ephraim and Menashe and said that in the future their names will be used as a blessing, and the people of Israel will say may 'God make you like Ephraim and Menashe'." (Genesis 48:20). Jacob's blessing on these two boys was that they should be a blessing, and an example to all Jewish children.

Parents traditionally recite this prayer for their children on Friday night as Shabbat begins. Some parents stand and place their hands on their child's head when they say the words. Then afterwards parents will often whisper a special prayer to their child saying something specific about them or their week ahead or thanking them for being good or doing well.

These are very special moments for children and their parents. It's a way of connecting with your child that is unlike many others and really differentiates relationships on Shabbat from other days of the week.

Here are the words of the Blessing of the Children:

For a girl:

יְשִׂימֵךְ אֱלֹהִים כְּשָׂרָה, רִבְקָה, רָחֵל וְלֵאָה.
Y'simeich Elohim k'Sarah, Rivkah, Rachel, v'Leah.
May you be like Sarah, Rebecca, Rachel, and Leah.

For a boy:

יְשִׂימְךָ אֱלֹהִים כְּאֶפְרַיִם וְכִמְנַשֶּׁה.
Y'simcha Elohim k'Efrayim v'chi-Menasheh.
May you be like Ephraim and Menashe.

For all:

יְבָרֶכְךָ אֲדֹנָי וְיִשְׁמְרֶךָ.

יָאֵר אֲדֹנָי פָּנָיו אֵלֶיךָ וִיחֻנֶּךָ.

יִשָּׂא אֲדֹנָי פָּנָיו אֵלֶיךָ וְיָשֵׂם לְךָ שָׁלוֹם.

Y'varechecha Adonai V'yish'm'recha.
Ya'er Adonai panav eilecha vichuneka.
Yisa Adonai panav eilecha v'yasem l'cha shalom.

May God bless you and guard you.
May God show you favor and be gracious to you.
May God show you kindness and grant you peace.

16.

Jewish Adoption:
Welcoming All Children into our Home

Not flesh of my flesh
Nor bone of my bone
But miraculously my own
Never forget for a minute
You didn't grow under my heart
But you grew in my heart!
B'rukha ha-ba'ah. We welcome you!
You are your parents' dreams realized, their hope fulfilled.
You are the latest and best chapter in the unfolding of the lives of your
Mother and Father
You are brand new—a symbol of today and tomorrow
Your life is a new and clean slate upon which people and events will
leave their impression.
You are a bridge over which we who welcome you can gaze from this
day into future days, from our generation into your generation.
You are the newest link in the endless chain of our people's history.
B'rukha haba'ah b'ahavah, we welcome you into the community of
the Jewish people—with love.

Welcoming a child into your home is one of the most loving, beautiful and fundamentally life-affirming acts. Judaism celebrates all children, no matter what type of journey they took into a Jewish home. Wherever a child was born, whatever the color of her skin is, she can be fully Jewish and embraced and loved by the Jewish community. In the following chapter I talk more about conversion, but here I want to give you an introduction to the roots and traditions

---

*Published with permission from "Naming Ceremony for an Adopted Child" originally published at *Ritualwell.org.*

of adoption in our Jewish culture.

Do Jewish couples adopt?

Yes! In fact, some studies suggest that Jewish families are more likely to adopt children than non-Jewish families. According to the U.S. Census Bureau's 2000 study, 2.5% of all American families have an adopted child in their family. In the National Jewish Population Study done that same year, over 5% of Jewish households reported having an adopted child in their home. Compared to the national average, Jewish families adopt at the rate of 2:1!

I spoke to Dr. Jayne Guberman & Jenny Sartori, the co-directors of the Adoption & Jewish Identity Project, and asked them what they thought explains this difference. Jenny told me that she thinks part of the reason is that many Jewish families "champion progressive values" and are willing to adopt across boundaries of identity (including children from other countries or who have a skin color different than their own). There are also socioeconomic factors involved; private and international adoptions are both very expensive and Jewish families are, on average, more able to afford these costs.

The modern day Hebrew word from adoption is אימוץ, pronounced *aimutz*. Jayne told me that the word *aimutz* is rooted in the Hebrew word for *graft*, as in a place on a tree where one branch has fallen off and a branch from a different tree grows together with it in that spot. Often the place where the graft takes hold is even stronger than the rest of the branch. This modern Hebrew word is significant in how it demonstrates very positive feelings toward the adoption process.

If adopting a child who has been born into a Jewish family already is important to you, that is also an option. Jewish children who are adopted by non-Jewish parents are likely to lose this component of their heritage; therefore some rabbis encourage Jewish parents to try to adopt these children first. There are also many Jewish children with special needs who are looking for permanent homes and families. If you are interested in learning more about this type of adoption, reach out to the Jewish Children's Adoption Network (jewishchildrensadoption.org) which facilitates them.

Jewish couples adopt, but is it acceptable under Jewish law?

"He who brings up a child is to be called its father, not he who gave birth."   —*Shemot Rabbah* 46:5

This quote is from the midrash associated with the book of Exodus. It was likely written during medieval times, but is a prominent example of the Jewish view of what makes someone a parent. In Judaism, it is considered a great mitzvah to adopt a child.

While there isn't a word for adoption in the Torah, there are many stories that include people who are welcomed into other families. One central story involves Abraham talking to God about his concern that he does not have offspring to inherit from him or to be his heir. In Genesis 15:2 Abraham says to God that since he is childless, his steward Eliezer shall be his heir. This is the first mention of how an adopted heir would deserve the same inheritance as a biological heir. It was also customary in Biblical times for the patriarch of the home to have children with his wife's maidservants (as experienced by Rachel and Sarah when they were unable to have children). In these cases, these children would be, in a way, adopted by the husband and wife and live as their own children.

Of course the most famous story of adoption in the Torah is really the story of the Torah itself. Also knows as the Five Books of Moses, the Torah is a story of a boy who was adopted. Moses was placed into the Nile River and adopted by Pharaoh's daughter and raised as an Egyptian.

Another famous adopted child in Jewish history is Queen Esther from the story of Purim. On the holiday of Purim we read the Megillah which begins with the background that Esther's parents had died, and so she was raised by her Uncle Mordechai.

In the book of Samuel there is a story about a woman named Michal who was unable to bear children, yet raised five sons with her husband David. The rabbinic commentary on this story is that the children were born to Michal's sister, but she raised them. This story is one of the main reasons rabbis conclude that a child's parents are the people who raise him, not give birth to him.

These historic references provide a fundamentally supportive historical context for Jewish families to pursue adoption knowing that according to Jewish law, their children must be welcomed and accepted.

In Judaism, lineage and parenthood play a big role in identity. For example, when you are called up to the Torah your name is announced as "son of So-and-So" or "daughter of So-and-So." This naming tradition is also used on your Wedding ketubah and any other time you are officially using your Jewish name. Your full Jewish name, therefore, has your parents' names built into it. In ancient times, Jewish people did not have surnames; they were just known by who their parents were. If someone does not know who their parents are, they use the term "son/daughter of Israel." But for someone who has been adopted, all the Jewish movements agree that they should use their adopted parents' names.

Where does identity come from?

Although adoption is officially accepted by Jewish law, there are, of course, challenges within the Jewish community for adopted children and their families. Adoptive parents worry that their children may experience feelings of being an outsider in a community that traditionally all looks the same.

Jenny and Jayne from the Adoption & Jewish Identity Project explained to me that one of the complexities of adoption today is that while past generations put an emphasis on religious and cultural matching in adoption, this is no longer standard policy in the U.S. As a result, the vast majority of kids who are adopted into Jewish homes were not born Jewish, so they are being brought up with their own identity as well as the complexities of a Jewish identity.

There are many Jewish organizations that offer workshops and advice on these topics. I recommend starting with the Adoption & Jewish Identity Project's Facebook group.

While any child may struggle with their identity as they grow up, Jewish communities today are becoming more diverse, inclusive, and welcoming of Jews who are different. However, we're not completely there yet, and there are still many moments in an adopted child's life when their uniqueness can cause confusion or pain. Jayne and Jenny have spent years researching what this reality has felt like for adopted children. They are releasing a new booklet called *18 Things Jewish Adoptive Kids Wish Their Parents and Communities Knew*, which tells these stories from the perspective of adopted kids in their own words.

I asked Rabbi Shira Stutman what her experience has been like counseling couples who are considering adoption. We talked about how sometimes there is a component of loss and sadness that comes with the realization that having a biological child isn't a possibility and the best option is to adopt. Though some couples seek out adoption first, or maybe after having a biological child, for those who come to this decision after years of infertility, there are sometimes mixed emotions. For Jewish families there can be an added element of identity struggles; if the child wasn't born Jewish, people want to know, are they still part of the *chosen people*? Rabbi Stutman reminded me that "People who convert are even holier than people born Jewish, because they chose it."

Joel Kushner, Director at the Kalsman Institute on Judaism and Health, shared his personal experience with adoption. He and his partner have two children: one who was born in Guatemala and one to whom his best friend gave birth. He told me that he always knew he wanted children, but wasn't sure exactly how that would come to fruition. He adopted his son at the age of four-and-a-half and worried whether he would feel like a "full parent" because of his son's age. Today he says that despite others making assumption or asking questions about his family, he feels fully and completely that his children are *his* children. For Joel, adopting a child meant fulfilling the core Jewish value that we care for people. In Judaism no one should go hungry while we have extra food; there is always a seat at the table; and no one in need, especially a child, should be abandoned.

Jewish kids are looking more and more diverse with each passing generation. In 2018, in a survey of freshmen in college, 20% of Jewish students identified as being Jews of color. Part of that number is Sephardic Jewish (about 10%) and the rest are Black, Asian, or mixed. If you're planning to adopt across race and ethnicity lines, Rabbi Stutman encourages couples she works with to seek out a welcoming synagogue and Hebrew School for them to attend.

Unfortunately we can't expect that every synagogue in America will be that place. It makes sense to tour these places in person and get a feel for the demographics of the congregation. Sending your child to Jewish day school as the *only* black Jewish kid there might be a difficult adjustment for them. It's not easy, but there are welcoming communities if you seek them out and advocate for your child when the time arises.

Rabbi Stutman is adamant that Judaism is "additive," that there is always room for inclusion. For example, today you can find Jewish Yoga Shabbat all over the U.S. When you think about it, this is not just combining an American fad with ancient Jewish ritual (which is part of the attraction); it's also borrowing from ancient Asian and Buddhist practices of meditation and physical restoration, to improve the Shabbat experience for the attendees. Every pocket of Judaism around the world has borrowed from their local culture to shape their Judaism. This is why Sephardi and Ashkenazi Jews have such different traditions.

Rabbi Stutman explained that there are ways to include the culture of your adopted child into Jewish practices. For example, if you adopted a baby from China, you could include some chopsticks on the Seder plate, or whatever item is meaningful to you and your family. As long as you do so with integrity and love it can increase the joy and meaning of the holiday. Jews have been adding to Judaism for thousands of years; some Jewish laws even been expanded to make observing their mitzvot more relatable for more people. Rabbi Avraham Kook, one of the most influential rabbis of the 20th century, was passionate about some of these aspects of Judaism. He taught that being inclusive and welcoming creates a community that is greater than the sum of its parts.

Naming ceremony for an adopted child

There are many options when it comes to celebrating a child being adopted into your family. To welcome a new baby or child to your Jewish community and synagogue, a naming ceremony (at any age!) can be a beautiful homecoming celebration. Your first stop can be your rabbi, to see if they have experience in this area and if they can help you plan something.

If you're looking for additional inspiration on what to do or say during the ceremony, check out *RitualWell.org*, which has lots of beautiful quotes and prayers to incorporate. Also, you can ask your synagogue about announcing the child's arrival to the family just as they would any other birth in the community. Many synagogues share adoption announcements along with birth announcements.

You can also include elements of your child's birth culture into the naming ceremony. For example, Jayne and Jenny told me about keeping a child's birth name to use as their middle name or another traditional name from that culture to use as a middle name. During the naming ceremony, you can talk about the name and its meaning. You can also say a traditional prayer from that birth culture, especially the child came from an international adoption and you want to preserve these components of your child's identity and be inclusive of their roots.

If you're participating in an open adoption you could invite the child's first parents to the naming ceremony and include them. It all depends on what your relationship and emotions are about this aspect of your child's beginnings. Jenny explained that even if a child's extended family isn't a part of your life, modern technology and culture are moving toward more openness and transparency—so you may want to embrace this spirit of inclusion from the outset.

Blessings over an adopted child

Here are some core components of the ceremony adapted from the website *RitualWell.org*, which provides many ideas for this celebrating this type of simcha. After welcoming guests and speaking about the child and her name you can include this adapted version of the Blessing over a Child from RitualWell:

יְשִׂמֵךְ אֱלֹהִים כְּשָׂרָה רִבְקָה רָחֵל וְלֵאָה

יְבָרֶךְ אֲדֹנָי וְיִשְׁמְרֶךְ

יָאֵר אֲדֹנָי פָּנָיו אֵלַיְךְ וִיחֻנֶּךְ

יִשָּׂא אֲדֹנָי פָּנָיו אֵלַיְךְ וַיָשֵׂם לָךְ שָׁלוֹם

Y'simekh elohim k'Sarah Rivkah Rakhel v'Leah
Y'varekh'kha Adonay v'yishm'rekha
Yaer Adonay panav elekha vikhunekha
Yisa Adonay panav elekha v'yasem l'kha shalom.

May God Make you like Sarah, Rebecca, Rachel and Leah.
May God bless you and keep you.
May God shine God's countenance unto you and be gracious to you
May God lift God's countenance to you and may God give you peace.

רִבּוֹן הָעוֹלָם בָּרֵךְ אֶת הַיַּלְדָּה הַזֹּאת בְּחַיִּים שֶׁל שִׂמְחָה חַיִּים שֶׁל טוֹבָה חַיִּים שֶׁל חָכְמָה. יְהִי רָצוֹן שֶׁתִּהְיֶה יַלְדָתֵנוּ עֹשָׂה שָׁלוֹם וְרוֹדֶפֶת שָׁלוֹם בֵּין אִישׁ לְרֵעֵהוּ. חַזֵּק יָדֵינוּ לְהַדְרִיכָהּ בְּדַרְכֵי תוֹרָה וֶאֱמוּנָה וְאַמְּצֵנוּ לְהוֹלִיכָהּ בְּעִקְבוֹת גְּבוּרוֹת יִשְׂרָאֵל שֶׁמַּעֲשֵׂיהֶם זָרְחוּ לָנוּ בְּכָל דּוֹרוֹת עַמֵּנוּ

Ribon ha-olam barekh et ha-yaldah hazot b'khayim shel simkhah khay-im shel tovah khayim shel khokhmah. Y'hi ratzon shetih'yeh yal'dat-eynu osah shalom v'rodefet shalom beyn ish l're'ehu. Khazek yadeynu l'hadrikhah b'darkhey torah ve'emunah v'amtzeynu liholikhah v'ikvot gibborot yisrael shema'aseyhem zarkhu lanu b'khol dorot ameynu.

Our God and God of our ancestors may the life of this child be one of happiness, goodness, and wisdom. Grant that she may seek peace and pursue an end to strife in the world. May she spread light on all who know her. May she study the Torah and find delight in it. May she follow the steps of other great leaders of Israel, whose deeds continue to shine across the span of time.

After reciting these prayers, it can be beautiful to then touch on the three core elements of what we wish for all Jewish children: that they may grow into a life of Torah, chuppah and *ma'asim tovim*. Torah means that they will learn Jewish tradition and keep the commandments holy. Chuppah means that they will find love and reach their wedding day. Ma'asim tovim means a life full of good deeds, a compassionate, caring and kind heart.

Then it is customary to conclude with the traditional blessing over the child and to say the Shehecheyanu prayer, thanking God for helping us to reach this blessed day.

17.

Conversion

What makes a baby Jewish?

If you are not Jewish, or if you have welcomed a baby into your home via adoption, it's time to think about whether or not to have an official conversion for your child. Jewish law holds that a baby is born Jewish if their mother is Jewish. This ancient tradition dates back to a time when determining paternity may have been impossible, so it made sense for religion to be passed down matrilineally. Spiritually speaking this is also a very empowering and beautiful concept—the mother shares her soul and her faith with her baby in the womb and they carry it with them when they are born.

Today there are many interfaith marriages, and many families have to determine how to proceed once they have a child. There are infinite pros and cons to either decision you make. Many couples are reluctant to choose at all, preferring that their child make their own decision when they are old enough to do so.

The Reform movement many years ago began accepting patrilineal descent, meaning that if the baby was born to a Jewish father and non-Jewish mother they would be considered Jewish and would not need to undergo the conversion process. The Conservative and Orthodox movements, however, would still require a conversion.

These specifics can be tricky and do change over time, so if you are considering conversion your first step should be to decide which movement in Judaism your family is most comfortable with. Will your child grow up in the Orthodox, Conservative, Reform or Reconstructionist movement? Once you are set on the community you would like your child to become a part of, then you can move forward with a rabbi who will take you along the conversion process. Each rabbi will have their own tailored instructions for how to proceed with the conversion but there are a few core components which all Jewish conversions have. The most significant of these is immersion in the mikvah, the final component to officially 'become' Jewish.

I personally have attended just one conversion of a baby relative of mine and I was totally wowed by the experience. Nothing in my 20ish years of spiritual life had been anything like it. I had attended Jewish day school, gone to Jewish summer camp and participated in all the Jewish holidays. Each had many wonderful and unique traditions—but nothing like immersing in the mikvah with a little baby to welcome them into a people and faith so longing to embrace them.

I remember most of all the mikvah attendant telling the parents to blow a quick breath right in front of the baby's face which would make them shut their eyes, and hold their nose as they went under the water for just a second. It was one of those moments when everyone in the room held their breath to see what would happen. There's no substance on Earth (in my opinion!) as beautiful, natural and spiritual as water, and it really was an honor to get to see a conversion ceremony in the mikvah.

To convert or not to convert: That's a really important question

Choosing your child's religion is undoubtedly an enormous decision. Choosing how to influence their faith, their relationship with God, and the people and culture to connect to their history can contribute to one of the most important parts of their identity. Or, an official conversion could just be a formal document that sits in a drawer and doesn't play much of a role in your child's life. Chances are though, if having a conversion for your child is important enough to go through, then it will be something meaningful and important throughout their life.

Of course only you and your partner can make this decision, but here are some helpful things to consider. If you decide not to convert your baby, you may encounter some tension if you'd like them to participate in religious schooling or Jewish summer camps; if you'd like them to become bar or bat mitzvah; if they would like to marry someone Jewish; and if they would like to go to Israel. That being said, there are many openly inclusive and welcoming Jewish communities who will work with you and your family to include your child even if he or she has not been officially converted to Judaism. For example, I grew up going to *Jewish* summer camp, but our director made it clear it was not a summer camp *only* for Jewish kids. Any child who wanted to attend was welcome. But not all communities are like that.

Lastly, some couples find it helpful to speak to other couples in similar situations about why they chose to make the decisions they did. These conversations elicit advice and give you new things to consider, but they can also bring up feelings and defensive instincts about your faith and your decisions that you might want to keep untriggered. Proceed with caution.

A Jewish conversion: how it works!

An incredibly helpful resource for grappling with these decisions and their ramifications is Anita Diamant's newly revised book, '*Choosing a Jewish Life: A Handbook for People Converting to Judaism and for Their Family and Friends*' which details the elements of conversion from choosing a rabbi to choosing a Hebrew name. The book also discusses how to have conversion discussions with family.

While the conversion ceremony for a baby or young child is quite simple, the most complicated component is deciding which type of conversion to have. The Orthodox, Conservative, Reconstructionist and Reform movements each have their own strict guidelines for what constitutes a kosher conversion.

Conversion is one aspect of Jewish religion that is very strict. This isn't one of those, *well, if you don't feel like keeping kosher, don't!* It's more of the *if you don't have an approved conversion ceremony you aren't a Jew* type thing (harsh, I know!). Some movements won't recognize a conversion performed by anyone other than their own. These same groups also do not recognize Jewish marriages that are not performed by their movement's rabbis. These politically divisive issues run deep and affect many components of the community. Generally though, an Orthodox conversion is the most widely accepted; but an Orthodox rabbi is unlikely to perform a conversion for a family who are not practicing Orthodox Jews.

It's best to speak with the rabbi of the synagogue you belong to or might become members of and ask them what conversion practices are accepted. Some require specific rabbis or institutions to perform the ceremony. A formal conversion ceremony requires that it be witnessed and approved by a *beit din* or Jewish court. This is a very formal name for the presence of three individuals, one of whom must be a rabbi, who are subject matter experts when it comes to conversion.

When a child is born to a mother who is not Jewish or is adopted by a Jewish family, they do not automatically become Jewish. Orthodox and Conservative rabbis require different elements for conversion, depending on the age of the child. Most babies go through a conversion ceremony, which is often a beautiful and spiritual experience where they receive a Hebrew name and then are immersed in the mikvah (Jewish ritual bath).

Baby boys will also have their brit milah (circumcision) if they have not had one yet. Some parents will give the baby a kosher bris eight days after they are born but a few months before they are converted to make the conversion process simpler. If the boy has already had a circumcision but it wasn't a kosher one some rabbis will require a mohel to perform a *hatafat dam brit*, where a tiny drop of blood is drawn from the penis before the baby is immersed in a mikvah. If you do not wish to circumcise your baby boy, you can speak to the rabbi about options for a *hatafat dam* and see what they recommend.

The immersion in the mikvah is often a beautiful and joyous ceremony where the mother and father go into the water with the baby to ensure their safety. Often they will place the baby just above the water and then let them into the water very gently before very quickly bringing them right back up as soon as their head goes beneath the surface. The actual time under the water can be just an instant. This ceremony is observed by the *beit din* mentioned earlier. In the Reform community the baby is only required to take a Hebrew name in addition to their English name; and for boys, to have had a circumcision. So if you decide to have a conversion with the Reform movement you will not need to go to the mikvah. If it is meaningful to you, discuss it with your rabbi.

Converting a baby without their knowledge is approved in Jewish law, as it is considered a privilege to be Jewish. However, many rabbis will also recommend that the child be informed of his conversion before his bar mitzvah, because he should be allowed to choose whether to accept it when he reaches maturity. At that point young adults can renounce their Judaism or choose to continue with their religious tradition.

Welcoming the convert

Many parents have anxiety about whether their child will be accepted in the Jewish community after their conversion. The good news is that Jewish tradition very specifically states that people who have converted must be welcomed. Our rabbis believe that God has a special love for people who convert, and that the people of Israel must bring God's love to the convert here in this world. Below are two quotes from ancient Jewish texts that speak to these principles:

God loves the righteous; God watches over the stranger (Psalm 146:8-9)

For I honor those who honor Me. (I Samuel 2:30)

Jewish people believe that God loves people who choose to be Jewish as a response to the love they show Him. There's a famous *midrash* (commentary) about people who choose Judaism. The story goes that a deer attaches himself to the King's flock. Every day the King tells his shepherd to take special care of this animal. When the shepherds ask him why, he responds that a lone animal who gives up the freedom of the wilderness to join the flock is a very special one that we should marvel at and appreciate. From this allegory the rabbis interpret that people who convert give up so much to abide by God's rules in the Torah and they honor our people's traditions by living a holy Jewish life. In the same way the King asked his shepherds to protect this deer, the Jewish people should go out of their way to protect and care for those who convert to Judaism.

18.

Random Advice and Funny Stories

Before we get into the actual useful bits of random advice, I'd like to share some of my favorite *un*helpful comments I hear from people. You probably won't be surprised to learn that strangers on the street start to interact with you a lot more once you have a kid, and they are liable to say the darndest things. It may have already begun; I know I got all sorts of comments once my pregnancy bump started showing.

I remember being asked by a cashier at a gas station convenience store if I was having twins because I looked so large (*nope!*), and the sales lady at Bloomingdale's asked if she could rub my belly for good luck (*uhh...sure?*). My son was born with a head of beautiful blonde curly hair but I have stick-straight brown hair, so we get asked almost daily where my son got his hair. At this point I just respond "the sperm donor" (which in fact is his dad!). Someone at synagogue once told me that our son's hair makes him "almost not look Jewish." And of course it's not just hair that strangers comment on, it's my mothering as well. At Trader Joe's I was told not to let him chew a toy he was teething on; at the mall I was told to put socks on his feet because he looked cold. *It. Never. Ends.* Now I get strangest feeling when I'm in public by myself because it feels like the world is ignoring me.

As I interviewed moms, rabbis and community leaders, I heard so many bits of actually *really* good advice on parenthood that I wanted to collect and share them with you here. If you prefer not to be told these types of things, I totally get it—read no further—but don't say I didn't try!

First, here's my personal best advice for new moms:

Newborns don't sleep; don't expect them to. If you can, try to accept the fact that—at least for the first little while—and come to terms with the reality that the only thing you'll have time and energy to do is take care of this new little person in your life. I don't know what I expected for the first few weeks of life with a newborn, but I didn't think that things like laundry and cooking dinner would become impossible tasks.

Try to let go of the feeling that you *need* to get stuff done while your baby is sleeping. You and your baby are linked; it took me a long time to learn to just let myself sleep when my baby did. Let go of the other things you wish you could be doing. I think for a lot of new moms this is the first prolonged break from a 40-hour workweek they've had since college, and they've dreamed of what they might do with this time.

Sure, you're going to take care of a baby, but you've been multi-tasking since kindergarten so you might think that your maternity leave will be a great time to redesign the kitchen and do every other home task you've always wished you had the luxury of time to enjoy doing. It is a huge shock to the system when you realize that this whole maternity leave thing exists because it's almost physically impossible to do much else besides take care of a newborn. A lot of that reality is because most babies don't sleep for more than a few hours at a time (definitely not at night!) and adults are not wired this way. I've found that if you give in for the first few weeks, you'll be much happier.

My other insider tip is that when it's time to transition to a schedule and you're going to attempt sleep training (always consult your pediatrician first; we started around 6 months), there really is only one method. You can Google all night long but in the end you'll realize that every sleep consultant, sleep book and sleep app all have the same core method. Babies need to learn to fall asleep on their own, it's a critical life skill that takes time and frustration for them to figure out and during this frustrating time they will cry. Whatever name or mnemonic you invest in, in the end it will mean the baby has to cry it out in some way. I share this because I spent many a long night trying to find an alternative. Aside from co-sleeping or giving up on the idea of a schedule and sleeping through the night altogether, the answer involves some tears.

And finally, YOU are the parent and YOU are in charge. Be a mama bear when you feel you need to and snuggle and cuddle whenever you want, You are the only mom (or parent) your kid will ever have, but every day is a second chance to be a better one.

Here is a collection of advice from some of the moms I interviewed for this book:

Rachel (children age 3,6,9)

"Sleep when the baby sleeps! And hydrate. Also, get your baby on a schedule, and let them cry it out."

Her funniest baby story—the first time she changed her baby boy's diaper and he peed all over the wall! (There are many funny peeing incidences when it comes to boys!)

Shira (children age 1, 4, 6)

"No one tries to give a mother having her third child advice! But the advice I give to others is to relax and don't get stressed comparing yourself to others. So your baby isn't the best sleeper—don't let someone else's sleep schedule make you feel like you're doing anything wrong."

Meg (children age 8, 8, 10)

Meg told me she actually tries not to give advice, because most of the time people really don't want to hear it! But her best advice is to "just to take it easy" and in your last month of pregnancy, try not to work yourself too hard especially right up until the end.

Sandra (children age 32, 39, 43)

"Drink black tea and have some crackers when you first wake up to stave off morning sickness." She says that anytime in her first trimester she was hungry she felt sick, so constant snacking really helped. And she actually recommends to stay busy and work up until the baby is born so as not to get anxious about the baby's arrival!

Katie (child age 1)

"The most helpful advice I got was to be gentle with myself. I wanted to keep doing everything I normally did! But I had one rough yoga class when I was about 11 weeks along, so I went to a prenatal yoga class the next week, and it changed my life. My teacher really instilled in me the idea that I was changing—physically, emotionally, spiritually—and that meant that I had to change the way I used my body while pregnant.

"The advice I give to expectant moms is to be gentle with themselves. I really encourage them to do prenatal yoga! I went every week from week 12 to 35. Then I went almost every day from week 35 until I gave birth at week 40. My yoga studio is a mile walk from my home, so it was a great way to stay active and social. The last time I went (which was three days before I gave birth), two expectant moms came up to me at the end of class and told me that I had inspired them to be more active. That really meant a lot to me, to know that I was helping other mamas! My other advice is to rent maternity clothes! I did and I loved it! It helped me feel cute all the way until the end."

Erin (child age newborn)

"I lost 8 pounds in the first 2 months from morning (all day) sickness. I was thrilled we were expecting as we had been trying for close to a year and had just been told we might need medical interventions. But I felt miserable, so there were multiple times I almost regretted it and struggled with the guilt of that. Thankfully other mothers told me not to feel guilty and to own every feeling I felt because they were all valid.

"Take every piece of advice with a grain of salt and know that most people are coming from a place of good intentions. You choose what's right for you and your family. Go with your gut!"

Rabbi Danielle Gobuty Eskow, President and Founder of OnlineJewishLearning.com (children age newborn, 2, 4)

"Be kind to yourself. This is the most difficult, amazing, exhausting time; but balloons, roses, love, and smiles help—, so does a good support system of friends. Don't expect things to go how they are in a movie, and don't let the difference between that and reality make you feel like something is wrong."

Tiffany, Instagram @raisingbumbles (children age 2 and 6)

"Follow your instincts! Advice from others is always good, if it's asked for, but it all comes down to you and your baby. If your instinct is telling you anything, follow it! And don't worry about what others think."

Beth (children age 29 and 32)

"Try to be relaxed and be present and in the moment."

Shawna (child age 4)

"Super cliché, but sleep when the baby sleeps. And be kind to yourself and take care of you. And know that when you feel like you're not doing a good job, it means you really care and you're doing great!!"

Stacey (child age 4)

"Trust yourself!"

Debbie (children age 31 and 35)

"My best advice is the age-old advice that everything will work itself out. Seek out family members and friends who you respect and collect advice from them. No one can force you to follow someone else's advice, but it's always helpful to hear other people's perspective on a situation similar to yours. It can also make you feel better that you are not the only one who has questions about a certain issue."

Miranda, public Instagram @Mirandahkemp (children age 1 and 3)

"Create a good support system for childcare and nurture adult relationships with supportive friends. When it's a tough moment, the best thing to do is breathe slowly and know that this moment will pass and things will get easier."

Acknowledgements

This book was made possible thanks to the contributions from the following individuals:

Maharat Ruth Balinsky Friedman, Ohev Shalom Synagogue, Washington, D.C.

Rabbi Nina Beth Cardin

Rabbi Sara Brandes, Executive Director at the Or HaLev: Center for Jewish Spirituality and Meditation; Shechinah Counsel, At the Well

Gila Block, Executive Director and Co-Founder of Yesh Tikva

Carrie Bornstein, Executive Director, Mayyim Hayyim

Rabbi Jaclyn Cohen, Temple Isaiah, West Los Angeles

Dalia Davis, President, Uprooted: A Jewish Response to Fertility Journeys

Anita Diamant, Author

Elana Frank, Executive Director and Founder of the Jewish Fertility Foundation

Rabbi Dara Frimmer, Temple Isaiah, West Los Angeles

Dr. Jayne Guberman & Jenny Sartori, co-Directors of the Adoption & Jewish Identity Project

Rabbi Danielle Gobuty Eskow, President and Founder of Online-JewishLearning.com

Rabbi and Doula Denise Handlarski of SecularSyngagogue.com

Hillary Kener, Director, National Outreach and Marketing at JScreen

Na'amah Wendy Kenin, the founding doula of Imeinu Doulas and Jewish Birth Collective

Joel Kushner, Director, Kalsman Institute on Judaism and Health

Dr. Lori Lefkovitz, PhD, Ruderman Professor of Jewish Studies and Humanities Center Director at Northeastern University

Rabbi Naomi Levy

Rabbi Myrna Matsa

Rabbi Idit Solomon, Founder and CEO of Hasidah

Rabbi Shira Stutman, Senior Rabbi, Sixth and I Synagogue Washington, D.C.

Sarah Waxman, Founder, At The Well

Rabbi Stuart Weinblatt, Temple Bnai Tzedek, Potomac Maryland

…and interviews with more than 50 real Jewish moms who have been through it all!

Additional Resources:

Jewish fertility support organizations:

Hasidah **hasidah.org** raises awareness and connects people to financial and other support resources in the Jewish community.

Jewish Fertility Foundation **www.jewishfertilityfoundation.org**

Mayyim Hayyim **mayyimhayyim.org**

PUAH Institute **puahonline.org** caters to the religious community, provides counseling and referrals free-of-charge, and has a board of rabbis to connect with couples.

Uprooted **weareuprooted.org/**

Yesh Tikva **yeshtikva.org**

Postpartum depression support:

National Suicide Prevention Help Line (1-800-273-8255)

NITZA - The Israel Center for Maternal Health caters to observant Jewish women in Israel **nitza.org**

Postpartum Education for Parents **sbpep.org**

Postpartum Support International **postpartum.net**

Delivery from Darkness: A Jewish Guide to Prevention, Detection and Treatment of Postpartum Depression by Rabbi Baruch Finkelstein, Michal Finkelstein, and Doreen Winter (Feldheim Publishers, 2009(

Waves of Blue: A Real-Life Experience With Postpartum Depression by Shoshanah Kagan (Israel Bookshop Publications: 2010).

Bibliography

All lines of text from Torah have been translated by sefaria.org

Amichai, Yehuda, Chana Bloch, and Stephen Mitchell. *The selected poetry of Yehuda Amichai.* Berkeley: University of California Press, 1996.

Artscroll Interlinear Siddur: The Schottenstein Edition. Brooklyn, NY: Artscroll Mesorah Publications, 2003.

Bialik, Mayim. "Mayim Bialik Talks About Sex." *Kveller,* https://www.kveller.com/mayim-bialik-talks-about-sex/

"Blessing the Children." My Jewish Learning. https://www.myjewishlearning.com/article/blessing-the-children/

Booth, David et al. "Modesty Inside and Out: A Contemporary Guide to Tzniut." Beth Tzedec Congregation Toronto. https://www.beth-tzedec.org/upload/media/1320/2017-teshuvah-modestyinsideandout.pdf

Clopper, Jeffrey. "Let's Fly Away...but not on Shabbes?" Temple Beth El of Huntington. July-August 2017 Bulletin. http://www.tbeli.org/wp-content/uploads/2017/06/July-August-2017-Bulletin.pdf

Falk, Sandy and Judson, Daniel. *The Jewish Pregnancy Book: A Resource for the Soul, Body & Mind during Pregnancy, Birth & the First Three Months.* Woodstock, VT: Jewish Lights Publishing, 2003.

Feinstein, Ed. "The Heart of Jewish Joy.'" *Jewish Journal.* https://jewishjournal.com/culture/religion/14502/

Frankel, Tamar. *The Voice of Sarah.* NY: HarperCollins, 1990.

"Immersion in the Mikveh." Mayyim Hayyim. https://www.mayyimhayyim.org/immersion-in-the-mikveh/

Friedman, Maharat Ruth. "When you're facing infertility, a synagogue can be the most painful place to go. Let's change that." *Washington Post.* https://www.washingtonpost.com/news/acts-of-faith/wp/2016/03/30/when-youre-facing-infertility-a-

synagogue-can-be-the-most-painful-place-to-go-lets-change-
that/?noredirect=on

Jacobson, Simon. "Marriage: Destiny or Chance." Chabad-Lubavitch
Media Center. https://www.chabad.org/theJewishWoman/article_
cdo/aid/600736/jewish/Marriage-Destiny-or-Chance.htm

"Jewish Parent/Child Relationships." My Jewish Learning, https://
www.myjewishlearning.com/article/jewish-parentchild-
relationships/

Paasche-Orlow, Rabbi Sara. "Acts of Loving-Kindness." My Jewish
Learning. https://www.myjewishlearning.com/article/acts-of-
loving-kindness/

"Pregnancy." Chabad-Lubavitch Media Center. https://www.chabad.
org/library/article_cdo/aid/690899/jewish/Pregnancy.htm

Rabin, Joshua. "Bedtime Shema." My Jewish Learning, https://www.
myjewishlearning.com/article/bedtime-shema/

"Shehecheyanu." Chabad-Lubavitch Media Center.
https://www.chabad.org/library/article_cdo/aid/91120/jewish/She-
hecheyanu.htm

"Shehecheyanu Prayer." Jewish Virtual Library. https://www.
jewishvirtuallibrary.org/shehecheyanu-blessing

Snir, Eleyor and Snir, Mirik. *When I First Held You: A Lullaby from
Israel*. Minneapolis, MN: Kar-Ben Publishing. 2009.

"Traditional Birkat Ha-Gomel." RitualWell. https://www.ritualwell.
org/ritual/traditional-birkat-ha-gomel

Wolfson, Ron. "How to Mourn Stillbirth and Neonatal Death."
My Jewish Learning. https://www.myjewishlearning.com/article/
stillbirth-and-neonatal-death/

"Vayeitzei: Marriage: Destiny or Chance?" Meaningful Life Center.
https://www.meaningfullife.com/vayeitzei-marriage-destiny-
chance/

"Views About Abortion." Pew Research Center.
https://www.pewforum.org/religious-landscape-study/views-about-
abortion/